Sports Endocrinology

Frontiers of Hormone Research

Vol. 47

Series Editor

Ezio Ghigo Turin

Co-Editor

Federica Guaraldi Turin

Sports Endocrinology

Volume Editors

Fabio Lanfranco Turin
Christian J. Strasburger Berlin

13 figures, 5 in color, and 13 tables, 2016

KARGER Basel · Freiburg · Paris · London · New York · Chennai · New Delhi · Bangkok · Beijing · Shanghai · Tokyo · Kuala Lumpur · Singapore · Sydney

Frontiers of Hormone Research
Founded 1972 by Tj.B. van Wimersma Greidanus, Utrecht
Continued by Ashley B. Grossman, Oxford (1996–2013)

Fabio Lanfranco, MD
Division of Endocrinology, Diabetology and Metabolism
Department for Medical Sciences
University of Turin
Turin (Italy)

Christian J. Strasburger, MD
Department of Medicine for Endocrinology, Diabetes and Nutritional Medicine
Charité Universitätsmedizin
Berlin (Germany)

Library of Congress Cataloging-in-Publication Data

Names: Lanfranco, Fabio, editor. | Strasburger, Christian J., editor.
Title: Sports endocrinology / volume editors, Fabio Lanfranco, Christian Strasburger.
Other titles: Sports endocrinology (Lanfranco) | Frontiers of hormone research ; v. 47. 0301-3073
Description: Basel ; New York : Karger, 2016. | Series: Frontiers of hormone research, ISSN 0301-3073 ; vol. 47 | Includes bibliographical references and indexes.
Identifiers: LCCN 2016018631| ISBN 9783318058680 (hard cover : alk. paper) | ISBN 9783318058697 (e-ISBN)
Subjects: | MESH: Sports--physiology | Endocrine Glands--physiology | Hormones--metabolism | Exercise--physiology | Physical Fitness--physiology | Doping in Sports
Classification: LCC QP571 | NLM QT 260 | DDC 612.4--dc23 LC record available at https://lccn.loc.gov/2016018631

Bibliographic Indices. This publication is listed in bibliographic services, including Current Contents® and PubMed/MEDLINE.

www.karger.com
Printed in Germany on acid-free and non-aging paper (ISO 9706) by Kraft Druck GmbH, Ettlingen
ISSN 0301–3073
e-ISSN 1662–3762
ISBN 978–3–318–05868–0
e-ISBN 978–3–318–05869–7

Contents

Foreword

In the last decades, the effects of physical activity on endocrine and metabolic functions have gained growing interest in the scientific world, not only among endocrinologists. On the other hand, the increasing availability of ergogenic aids and supplements for professional athletes and amateurs on the market has galvanized the debate on the potential short- and long-term positive and negative consequences of these substances.

Indeed, the pivotal role exerted by hormones and other peptides with paracrine and endocrine action on body homeostasis (in both basal and stressful conditions) and physical performance (through the modulation of both resistance and endurance) is well known. On the other hand, both acute and chronic exercise have important effects on the functioning of several organs and systems, mainly mediated by the endocrine and neuroendocrine system.

Not only a multitude of environmental factors, including dietary practices for both macronutrients and supplements, but also training characteristics (i.e. intensity, time of day, and duration), age, gender, and circadian hormone secretion patterns have a strong impact on the interactions between exercise and endocrine function.

This volume of the series *Frontiers of Hormone Research* provides an authoritative overview on the most innovative, and sometimes still debated, topics in sports endocrinology. The first section of this volume explores the effects of physical activity on endocrine and metabolic functions in relation to exercise performance, growth, development, and aging. The second section presents the main characteristics and effects of performance-enhancing endocrine drugs, as well as techniques for their detection.

We are proud to present Fabio Lanfranco and Christian J. Strasburger's book entitled *Sports Endocrinology*, both of them experts in the field. We truly believe that this book will be attractive and useful for endocrinologists as well as physicians, physiologists, pharmacologists, and internists involved in the field of sports medicine, and we are grateful to all contributors that have made this volume what it is.

Ezio Ghigo, Turin
Federica Guaraldi, Turin

Preface

Physical activity exerts an important influence on the endocrine system, modulating synthesis and secretion of several hormones. Almost every organ and system in the body is affected by physical activity and exercise, mainly through the endocrine and neuroendocrine system. Mode, intensity, and duration of the exercise bout, gender, age, and fitness level of the individual, as well as environmental and psychological factors may affect the endocrine response to physical activity.

In this book, the effects of physical activity and training on the endocrine function are extensively discussed and related to exercise performance, growth, development, and aging. A substantial part of this volume is devoted to the 'hot topic' of hormonal doping in sports. During the past decades, hormone abuse has become a widespread habit among professional and recreational athletes. The properties of androgens, growth hormone, erythropoietin as well as dietary supplements and their use and misuse in sports are described. Specific methods to detect hormone abuse are presented and discussed.

The contributors to this volume are well-known experts in the fields of sports medicine and endocrinology, endocrine physiology, pharmacology, and doping detection.

The purpose of this volume is to provide all professionals involved in sports medicine and endocrinology a state-of-the-art overview of the complex interactions between physical activity and the endocrine system and to focus on hormone use and abuse in sports at competitive and recreational level, highlighting its negative long-term consequences for health.

Fabio Lanfranco, Turin
Christian J. Strasburger, Berlin

Lanfranco F, Strasburger CJ (eds): Sports Endocrinology.
Front Horm Res. Basel, Karger, 2016, vol 47, pp 1–11 (DOI: 10.1159/000445147)

Growth Hormone-Insulin-Like Growth Factor Axis, Thyroid Axis, Prolactin, and Exercise

Anthony C. Hackney[a–c] · Hope C. Davis[b] · Amy R. Lane[b, c]

[a]Department of Nutrition – Gillings School of Global Public Health, [b]Department of Exercise and Sport Science, and [c]Human Movement Science Curriculum, University of North Carolina, Chapel Hill, N.C., USA

Abstract

This chapter addresses what is known about the endocrine system components growth hormone (GH)-insulin-like growth factor (IGF) axis, thyroid axis, and prolactin relative to exercise and exercise training. Each one of these hormone axes contributes to the maintenance of homeostasis in the body through impact on a multitude of physiological systems. The homeostatic disruption of exercise causes differing responses in each hormone axis. GH levels increase with sufficient stimulation, and IGFs are released in response to GH from the anterior pituitary providing multiple roles including anabolic properties. Changes in the thyroid hormones T_3 and T_4 vary greatly with exercise, from increases/decreases to no change in levels across different exercise types, intensities and durations. These ambiguous findings could be due to numerous confounding factors (e.g. nutrition status) within the research. Prolactin increases proportionally to the intensity of the exercise. The magnitude may be augmented with extended durations; conflicting findings have been reported with resistance training. While the responses to exercise vary, it appears there may be overall adaptive and regenerative impacts on the body into recovery by these hormones through immune and tissue inflammatory responses/mediations. Nonetheless, well-designed exercise research studies are still needed on each of these hormones, especially thyroid hormones and prolactin.

The endocrine system consists of a series of glandular tissues located throughout the human body, which secrete hormones to serve as chemical messengers that can modify and regulate the physiological function of tissues. Numerous hormones not only have such 'endocrine-like' effects, but also have 'autocrine' and 'paracrine' functions, which collectively allow for these substances to have far-reaching and powerful physiological effects. Additionally, recent discoveries point to many nonglandular tissues in the human body that secrete hormones and hormone-like substances (e.g. cytokines from skeletal muscles).

Such discoveries have added to the complexity of trying to understand the endocrine-hormone interactive controls involved when the homeostasis of the body is challenged. A potent disruptor to the homeostasis of the body is physical exercise and exercise training. Numerous research studies have quantified the dynamic and robust hormonal responses to exercise activities, whether these activities involve cardiovascular function for prolonged periods (endurance) or skeletal muscle strength-power in an explosive nature (resistance).

The purpose of this article is to provide a concise discussion on the current understanding of the roles of the pituitary hormones prolactin and growth hormone (GH), the insulin-like growth factor (IGF)-GH axis, and the thyroid axis with respect to physical exercise and exercise training. Contemporary endocrinology research points to interactive roles for the specific hormones associated with these axes and glands, which play key physiological roles with respect to effects on the ability to do physical exercise and the adaptation process following exercise training.

Growth Hormone-Insulin-Like Growth Factor Axis

GH is a family of hormones with over 100 variants in isoform and aggregate combinations [1, 2]. The isoform that is most common and typically measured in most exercise studies is the 191-amino acid (22-kDa) variant. This 22-kDa form will be the focus of this discussion here within when referring to GH. The specific role of each variant (isoform or aggregate) is yet to be fully determined as far more research is needed, but exercise does appear to be an effective stimulator for the production and release of many of these variants, i.e. acute increases can be observed following single exercise bouts as well as chronic elevations in response to select exercise training programs [3].

Regulation

Relative to regulation, in response to an exercise bout, GH-releasing hormone (GHRH) is secreted from the hypothalamus. GHRH travels along the hypophyseal portal vascular system to the anterior pituitary where GHRH receptor activation results in GH production/release from the somatotropic cells of the pituitary. In contrast, inhibition of GH production occurs due to the release of somatostatin (GH-inhibiting hormone). The key factors that influence the release of GHRH and GH-inhibiting hormone in this complex system are depicted in figure 1.

Exercise Effects

Increased circulation of GH is observed with exercise provided the amount of muscle mass recruited is great enough or there is a sufficient metabolic need [4, 5]. Furthermore, GH is very sensitive to changes in pH, as illustrated by a general direct relationship between blood lactate and GH with exercise [1]. For this latter reason, exercise

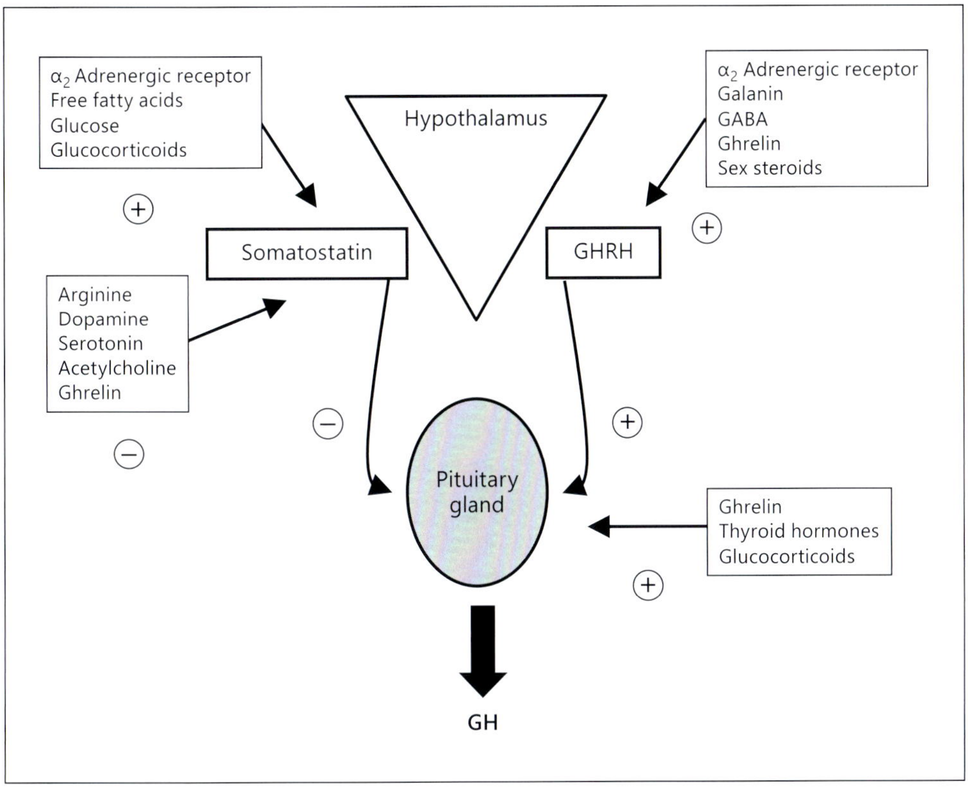

Fig. 1. Major factors involved with GH regulation at the hypothalamic-pituitary level.

sessions with protocols that challenge the acid-base/pH status (i.e. short rest-work cycles) can provoke dramatic GH increases [6–8].

Once released in the circulation, GH can exhibit pleiotropic effects, and it can play key roles in promoting increased lipid metabolism, chronological growth, reproduction, and immune and neural functions. Relative to endurance exercise and energy metabolism, the role of GH in lipid metabolism can be especially critical [1, 2]. In the context of exercise training (primarily strength or resistance based), GH also plays an important role in muscular development by select direct anabolic effects as well as by mediating circulating or locally produced IGF [9, 10].

Insulin-like Growth Factors

IGFs are hormone substances with structures similar to insulin and are very powerful anabolic substances. The IGF superfamily consists primarily of two cell surface receptors (IGF1R and IGF2R), two ligands IGF-1 and IGF-2, a group of six high-affinity IGF-binding proteins (IGFBP-1 to IGFBP-6), and associated IGFBP degrading enzymes, referred to collectively as proteases. The signal for the release of IGF is initiated by GH release at the anterior pituitary followed by a production and release of

IGF-1 from the liver [1, 10]. IGF-1 is considered a very important biomarker for health, fitness, and well-being [11].

Research has identified IGF-1 as the signal molecule for two essential intracellular cascades: mitogen-activated protein kinase (MAPK) and phosphatidylinositol 3-kinase (PI3K). IGF-2 appears to play more of a role in embryogenesis [12]. Interestingly, IGF-1 has shown variable responsiveness to resistance exercise, and the starting concentrations appear to be a major determinant if increases with an exercise stimulus (stress) are observed [13, 14]. With exercise training, increases in resting IGF-1 concentrations occur, which play an important role in the maintenance of physiological homeostasis [15].

Insulin-Like Growth Factor Binding Proteins and Receptors

In the circulation, IGF-1 is bound to one of six binding proteins. These binding proteins have roles in transporting IGF-1 to the target tissue [16]. Furthermore, there is evidence to suggest that the changes in these binding proteins (within the context of an exercise bout or training) are a critical aspect of modulating the bioactivity of IGF-1 [17–19]. Physiologically, it appears that it is not the amount of IGF-1 that is central, but the manner in which IGF-1 is segregated among its binding proteins [19].

IGF1R contains two extracellular α-subunits and two transmembrane β-subunits. IGF-1 binds to the α-subunits and induces autophosphorylation of the β-subunit. The mechanism of downstream signaling of the MAPK and PI3K cascades is determined by the interactions involving the insulin receptor substrate 1 [1, 15]. The MAPK cascade is primarily responsible for the proliferation of muscle cells. This occurs with increased expression in the amount and activity of transcription factors such as cyclins, D1, and D2 [20]. Cyclins are a family of proteins that control the progression of cells through the cell cycle by activating cyclin-dependent kinase enzyme while D1 and D2 are responsible for accelerating cell cycle progression [20]. The mitogenic activity of this pathway occurs essentially through the phosphorylation of extracellular signal-regulated kinases (i.e. ERK 1/2) which allows for cell proliferation [21]. Additionally, the PI3K cascade primarily mediates cell differentiation. PI3K signaling has three crucial roles: fusion of myoblasts into myotubes, anabolic effects on protein and glucose uptake, and resistance to apoptosis development [22].

Thyroid Axis

The thyroid is a critical endocrine gland in the human body. It produces and secretes three hormones: thyroxine [T_4 (3,5,3′,5′-tetraiodothyronine)], triiodothyronine [T_3 (3,5,3′-triiodothyronine)] and calcitonin. Both T_3 and T_4 are considered critical for the normal physiological function of a broad spectrum of tissues and organs due to their ability to modulate metabolism, and act synergistically with other hormones (i.e.

pleiotropic and permissive actions). Conversely, calcitonin is a key regulator in maintaining the circulating levels of calcium via the influence on osteoblastic cellular activity. For this discussion only, the role of T_4 and T_3 (collectively referred to as the 'thyroids') are addressed.

Regulation

The production and secretion of the thyroids is controlled by thyroid-stimulating hormone (TSH; also called thyrotropin), a glycoprotein-based hormone released from the adenohypophysis (anterior pituitary). Thyroid-releasing hormone (TRH) produced by the hypothalamus stimulates the release of TSH. The control and release of these hormones involve a negative feedback loop referred to as the hypothalamic-pituitary-thyroidal axis [23].

Once in the circulation, these hormones exist in a bound as well as in a free, unbound form. The carrier proteins for the bound forms of the hormones are thyroid-binding globulin (accounting for 70%), thyroxine-binding pre-albumin (10–15%), and albumin (15–20%). The unbound free forms of the hormones are a relatively small amount of each hormone's respective total amounts (free T_4 ~0.03% and free T_3 ~0.3%). These free forms are the most effective and biologically active versions of each hormone.

Circulating concentrations of T_4 exceed that of T_3, but T_3 is the more biologically potent of the hormones. The turnover rate of the thyroids is very low relative to their existing large extracellular hormonal pool. This fact can make it complex and challenging for researchers to detect hormonal changes, even relatively large ones, in thyroid gland activity following a disruption in homeostasis [23].

Most tissues are strongly influenced metabolically by the thyroids, and these hormonal changes can profoundly influence many tissue functions, growth, and development across the human age span [23–25]. As an illustration, thyroids increase oxidative phosphorylation in mitochondria and responsiveness to catecholamines (which can influence metabolic rate), and have a cardiogenic effect. A similar synergetic effect occurs for GH. The thyroids can augment all aspects of lipid metabolism in the body, especially within skeletal muscles. They also enhance hepatic glycogenolysis and influence protein degradation.

Exercise Effects

Short-term incremental exercise (<20 min) elevates TSH concentrations, with a critical intensity [oxygen uptake (VO_{2max})] threshold of approximately 50% of VO_{2max} being necessary to induce significant changes in the concentration [25, 26]. Even though TSH is elevated, most research on such short-term exercise indicates the concentrations of total and free T_4 and T_3 are not affected [25]. Reports of increases in total levels of thyroids during the recovery from such exercise exist; however, these findings appear to be the function of exercise hemoconcentration of the blood. An increase in TSH levels might be expected to stimulate the thyroid gland, but physiologically there is a delay inherent in the stimulus-secretion response of the gland [23]. Thus, if the blood sampling protocol was for a too short period of time (only a few hours) it would be expected that studies report the thyroids essentially unchanged by a single exercise session [24, 27, 28]. This limitation in methodology seems to exist in many exercise research studies.

Research findings in many situations are confounded, i.e. the influence of environmental factors, dietary practices, and diurnal hormonal secretion patterns were not controlled for effectively, and, therefore, they cannot be entirely separated from the influence of exercise alone. Also, it is unclear if observed exercise-induced changes in thyroids are in part due to changes in the concentrations of binding proteins. Although work on hormonal binding proteins in general suggests for most exercise, the free hormonal changes typically exceed the binding protein effects alone [24].

The influence of more prolonged exercise (>1 h) on thyroids is controversial as well. Several investigations found no effect on TSH levels in the blood [24, 26, 28] while others found TSH to increase progressively with high-intensity workloads and to reach an elevated steady-state level after approximately 40 min of exercise [24, 26]. As previously mentioned, an increase in TSH might be expected to cause an increase in T_4 or T_3, but physiologically the issue is complicated by the delayed response of the gland to a TSH stimulus [23].

Berchtold et al. [30] reported that during very prolonged submaximal exercise (~3 h), total T_4 remained constant but then declined significantly during recovery. In the same study, the level of T_3 continuously declined during exercise. Others, however, found total T_3 to remain unchanged but total T_4 to be increased by 60 min into a prolonged submaximal exercise session [27]. Galbo [27] showed strenuous, prolonged exercise to increase only free T_4 concentration. These divergent findings are difficult to interpret due to the highly varying duration intensities of exercise and blood sampling protocols used in these various studies.

Intensive single anaerobic exercise bouts (cycling) increase T_4 levels for several hours during the recovery from such exercise [27]. Regrettably, research on the effects of resistance exercise on thyroid hormones is sparse and suffers from some limitations. McMurray et al. [28] performed a well-controlled study assessing thyroid responses immediately after an intensive resistance training session, as well as for 12 h into recovery (during nighttime). Significant elevations in T_4 and T_3 were seen immediately after exercise, apparently primarily related to hemoconcentration [29]. Later, significant nocturnal elevations in T_3 levels were observed. Physiologically, the elevation in T_3 levels suggests that during recovery from resistance exercise there is an increase in metabolism, most likely associated with tissue repair [23].

Research findings on the effects of training programs on thyroids are ambiguous. Some studies, but not all, show the rate of T_4 secretion is higher in exercise-trained individuals than in untrained individuals [24, 26]. Conversely, Galbo [27] reported that short-term, intensive exercise training periods result in significant reductions in thyroid hormones. Basal and TRH-stimulated blood TSH responses were reported as similar in trained and sedentary humans [24]. The discrepancy in these findings may be related to the fact that these studies failed to completely account for the influence of nutrient balance on the thyroid turnover rate, i.e. a negative energy balance has been shown to substantially reduce the thyroid responses [23, 30–39]. However, Baylor and Hackney [35] followed elite athletes during a 20-week training competition cycle and found that resting free T_3 and TSH were reduced during intensive competitive periods even though no significant changes in body mass occurred. The turnover rate of thyroid hormones appears to increase in training athletes [24, 30, 37]. It is possible that the tissue sensitivity to T_3 [23, 30] could account for the free T_3 reduction noted above.

Prolactin

The hormone prolactin is primarily produced and secreted by lactotrope cells of the anterior pituitary, but there are also extrapituitary sources of the hormone – the breast, decidua, adipose tissue, parts of the central nervous system, and select immune system cells. Since it is released by extrapituitary sites, it is not only classified as a circulating hormone but also as an autocrine and paracrine factor. Many tissues within humans express prolactin receptors as it is a multifunctional hormone. For example, its release and subsequent function has been linked to emotional-physical stress, water balance regulation, fetal surfactant development, immune system activation, and reproductive function. Most published research on prolactin relates to this last topic because prolactin has long been associated with lactogenesis in women and gonadal suppression (at excessive circulating levels) in both men and women.

Regulation

In the circulation, prolactin displays a diurnal secretion pattern with peak levels during REM sleep at night [40]. There are a multitude of external and internal stimuli that influence hypothalamic neurons to secrete prolactin-releasing (PRFs) and -inhibiting factors (PIFs). PIFs or PRFs in turn affect the lactotrope cell production of prolactin. Prolactin is secreted in episodes, which is under inhibitory control exerted by dopamine as the main PIF. Stimulatory mechanisms for prolactin secretion result from the disinhibition of dopamine activity or superimposition of stimulatory input through one or more PRFs. There are several PRFs, including TRH, arginine vasopressin, vasoactive intestinal peptide, oxytocin, estrogen, pituitary adenylate cyclase-activating polypeptide, endogenous opioids, bradykinin, and substance P [40, 41].

Exercise Effects

Circulating prolactin concentrations increase with exercise, and the magnitude of the increase is approximately proportional to the intensity of the exercise activity. Whether there is a critical intensity threshold necessary to induce a hormonal response is uncertain, but most exercise above the anaerobic threshold initiates substantial increases [25, 27, 42]. Provided the intensity of exercise is appropriate, the increase in prolactin is quite rapid. However, short-term incremental exercise may result in a peak response occurring after the end of the exercise. In some situations, such as competitive sports, excessive emotional stress can cause an anticipatory increase in prolactin even before the initiation of exercise [25].

In a prolonged exercise session, the prolactin response is proportional to the intensity at which it is performed. However, extending the duration of exercise can augment the magnitude of the prolactin response [43, 44]. This change in prolactin seems to be strongly driven by the elevation in core temperature during the exercise [45]. For example, just the act of head-facial cooling has been shown to reduce the prolactin response of exercise to some degree [46]. Interestingly, after daytime sessions of prolonged exercise, there is an increase in the nocturnal levels of the hormone [47].

Vigorous, high-intensity anaerobic exercise (i.e. interval training) results in greater prolactin response than typically seen in submaximal steady-state aerobic exercise [48]. The effect of resistance exercise, which is intermittent in nature, on prolactin has not been extensively studied. Some evidence supports that this form of exercise will elevate prolactin, but the increase may occur sometime after the exercise session is completed [25]. Data are conflicting with regard to the chronic effect of exercise training on resting (basal) prolactin levels [49, 50]. These contradictions are most likely related to differences in training protocols (intensity, frequency, and duration of training sessions). Some researchers have shown that the prolactin response to submaximal exercise in men is attenuated following training, but the maximal exercise response is augmented [25, 51]. Interestingly, in both men and women who have undergone a training program, the drug-stimulated prolactin response is enhanced (i.e. pituitary challenge tests [52, 53]).

Interaction of the Hormones

The GH-IGF, thyroids, and prolactin are interconnected, as they share certain aspects of regulation in common. A prime example of this is the fact that an increase in TRH release from the hypothalamus is not only a stimulant to the release of TSH, but also to the release of pituitary GH and prolactin. In addition, sex steroids (e.g. estrogens) provide a regulatory link by also exerting a positive effect on GH, thyroids, and prolactin. Likewise, 'stressful' situations can result in TRH/TSH release as well as GH and prolactin release proportional to the magnitude of the stress [24, 40, 54].

Functionally, these hormonal interrelated responses during exercise can provide a multitude of beneficial physiological effects. For example, GH, IGFs, thyroids, and prolactin can be described, in general, as immune-permissive and immune-regulatory hormones [40, 55]. These hormones are associated with activities such as chemotaxis, phagocytosis, microbicidal capacity of phagocytes, cytokine production, and macrophage function [55]. Collectively, such functions-actions suggest that these hormones have potential roles, in concert, to aid and support the immune and tissue inflammatory responses after exercise as part of the adaptive-regeneration process with exercise and exercise training [41, 56]. Nonetheless, additional exercise research is needed to address this issue in detail and study the specifics of these interesting hormonal interactions.

References

1 Baumann G: Growth hormone heterogeneity: genes, isohormones, variants, and binding proteins. Endocr Rev 1991;12:424–449.

2 Kraemer WJ, Dunn-Lewis C, Comstock BA, Thomas GA, Clark JE, Nindl BC: Growth hormone, exercise, and athletic performance: a continued evolution of complexity. Curr Sports Med Rep 2010;9:242–252.

3 Kraemer WJ, Nindl BC, Marx JO, Gotshalk LA, Bush JA, Welsch JR, Volek JS, Spiering BA, Maresh CM, Mastro AM, Hymer WC: Chronic resistance training in women potentiates growth hormone in vivo bioactivity: characterization of molecular mass variants. Am J Physiol Endocrinol Metab 2006;291: E1177–E1187.

4 Milner-Brown HS, Stein RB, Yemm R: The orderly recruitment of human motor units during voluntary isometric contractions. J Physiol 1973;230:359–370.

5 French DN, Kraemer WJ, Volek JS, Spiering BA, Judelson DA, Hoffman JR, Maresh CM: Anticipatory responses of catecholamines on muscle force production. J Appl Physiol 2007;102:94–102.

6 Kraemer WJ, Fleck SJ, Dziados JE, Harman EA, Marchitelli LJ, Gordon SE, Mello R, Frykman PN, Koziris LP, Triplett NT: Changes in hormonal concentrations after different heavy-resistance exercise protocols in women. J Appl Physiol 1993;75:594–604.

7 Kraemer WJ, Marchitelli L, Gordon SE, Harman E, Dziados JE, Mello R, Frykman P, McCurry D, Fleck SJ: Hormonal and growth factor responses to heavy resistance exercise protocols. J Appl Physiol 1990;69: 1442–1450.

8 Hymer WC, Kraemer WJ, Nindl BC, Marx JO, Ben son DE, Welsch JR, Mazzetti SA, Volek JS, Deaver DR: Characteristics of circulating growth hormone in women after acute heavy resistance exercise. Am J Physiol Endocrinol Metab 2001;281:E878–E887.

9 Sotiropoulos A, Ohanna M, Kedzia C, Menon RK, Kopchick JJ, Kelly PA, Pende M: Growth hormone promotes skeletal muscle cell fusion independent of insulin-like growth factor 1 up-regulation. Proc Natl Acad Sci USA 2006;103:7315–7320.

10 Perrini S, Laviola L, Carreira MC, Cignarelli A, Natalicchio A, Giorgino F: The GH/IGF1 axis and signaling pathways in the muscle and bone: mechanisms underlying age-related skeletal muscle wasting and osteoporosis. J Endocrinol 2010;205:201–210.

11 Nindl BC, Pierce JR: Insulin-like growth factor I as a biomarker of health, fitness, and training status. Med Sci Sports Exerc 2010;42:39–49.

12 Frasca F, Pandini G, Scalia P, Sciacca L, Mineo R, Costantino A, Goldfine ID, Belfiore A, Vigneri R: Insulin receptor isoform A, a newly recognized, high-affinity insulin-like growth factor II receptor in fetal and cancer cells. Mol Cell Biol 1999;19:3278–3288.

13 Kraemer WJ, Marchitelli L, Gordon SE, Harman E, Dziados JE, Mello R, Frykman P, McCurry D, Fleck SJ: Hormonal and growth factor responses to heavy resistance exercise protocols. J Appl Physiol 1990;69: 1442–1450.

14 Kraemer WJ, Gordon SE, Fleck SJ, Marchitelli LJ, Mello R, Dziados JE, Friedl K, Harman E, Maresh C, Fry AC: Endogenous anabolic hormonal and growth factor responses to heavy resistance exercise in males and females. Int J Sports Med 1991;12:228–235.

15 Rubin MR, Kraemer WJ, Maresh CM, Volek JS, Ratamess NA, Vanheest JL, Silvestre R, French DN, Sharman MJ, Judelson DA, Gomez AL, Vescovi JD, Hymer WC: High-affinity growth hormone binding protein and acute heavy resistance exercise. Med Sci Sports Exerc 2005;37:395–403.

16 Nindl BC, Pierce JR: Insulin-like growth factor I as a biomarker of health, fitness, and training status. Med Sci Sports Exerc 2010;42:39–49.

17 Nindl BC, Alemany JA, Tuckow AP, Kellogg MD, Sharp MA, Patton JF: Effects of exercise mode and duration on 24-h IGF-I system recovery responses. Med Sci Sports Exerc 2009;41:1261–1270.

18 Nindl BC, Castellani JW, Young AJ, Patton JF, Khosravi MJ, Diamandi A, Montain SJ: Differential responses of IGF-I molecular complexes to military operational field training. J Appl Physiol 2003;95: 1083–1089.
19 Nindl BC, Kraemer WJ, Marx JO, Arciero PJ, Dohi K, Kellogg MD, Loomis GA: Overnight responses of the circulating IGF-I system after acute, heavy-resistance exercise. J Appl Physiol 2001;90:1319–1326.
20 Coolican SA, Samuel DS, Ewton DZ, McWade FJ, Florini JR: The mitogenic and myogenic actions of insulin-like growth factors utilize distinct signaling pathways. J Biol Chem 1997;272:6653–6662.
21 Fuentes EN, Bjornsson BT, Valdes JA, Einarsdottir IE, Lorca B, Alvarez M, Molina A: IGF-I/PI3K/Akt and IGF-I/MAPK/ERK pathways in vivo in skeletal muscle are regulated by nutrition and contribute to somatic growth in the fine flounder. Am J Physiol Regul Integr Comp Physiol 2011;300:R1532–R1542.
22 Singleton JR, Feldman EL: Insulin-like growth factor-I in muscle metabolism and myotherapies. Neurobiol Dis 2001;8:541–554.
23 Griffin JE: The thyroid; in Griffin JE, Odjeda SR (eds): Textbook of Endocrine Physiology, ed 3. New York, Oxford University, 1996, pp 260–283.
24 Mazzaferri EL: The thyroid; in Mazzaferri, EL (ed): Endocrinology, ed 3. New York, Medical Examination Publishing, 1985, pp 89–350.
25 McMurray RG, Hackney AC: The endocrine system and exercise; in Garrett WE, Kirkendall DT (eds): Exercise and Sports Science. New York, Williams & Wilkins, 2000, pp 135–162.
26 McMurray RG, Hackney AC: Interactions of metabolic hormones, adipose tissue and exercise. Sports Med 2005;35:393–412.
27 Galbo H: The hormonal response to exercise. Diabetes Metab Rev 1986;1:385–408.
28 McMurray RG, Eubanks TE, Hackney AC: Nocturnal hormonal responses to weight training exercise. Eur J Appl Physiol 1995;72:121–126.
29 Hackney AC, Viru A: Research methodology: endocrinologic measurements in exercise science and sports medicine. J Athl Train 2008;43:631–639.
30 Berchtold PM, Berger M, Uppers HJ: Non-glucoregulatory hormones (T4, T3, rT3, testosterone) during physical exercise in juvenile type diabetes. Horm Metab Res 1978;10:269–273.
31 Moore AW, Timmerman S, Brownlee KK, Rubin DA, Hackney AC: Strenuous, fatiguing exercise: relationship of cortisol to circulating thyroid hormones. Int J Endocrinol Metab 2005;3:18–24.
32 Hackney AC, Gulledge TP: Thyroid responses during an 8-hour period following aerobic and anaerobic exercise. Physiol Res 1994;43:1–5.
33 Opstad K: Circadian rhythm of hormones is extinguished during prolonged physical stress, sleep and energy deficiency in young men. Eur J Endocrinol 1994;131:56–66.
34 Irvine CHG: Effect of exercise on thyroxine degradation in athletes and non-athletes. J Clin Endocrinol Metab 1968;28:942–948.
35 Baylor LS, Hackney AC: Resting thyroid and leptin hormone changes in women following intense, prolonged exercise training. Eur J Appl Physiol 2003;88: 480–484.
36 Douyon L, Schteingart DE: Effect of obesity and starvation on thyroid hormone, growth hormone, and cortisol secretion. Endocrinol Metab Clin North Am 2002;31:173–189.
37 Balsam A, Leppo LE: Effect of physical training on the metabolism of thyroid hormones in man. J Appl Physiol 1975;38:212–215.
38 Terjung RL, Winder WW: Exercise and thyroid function. Med Sci Sports 1974;7:20–26.
39 DeNayer P, Ostyn M, DeVisscher M: Effet de l'entraînement sur le taux de la thyroxine libre chez l'athlète. AnnEndocrinol (Paris) 1970;31:721–723.
40 Ben-Jonathan N, Hugo ER, Brandebourg TG, LaPensee CR: Focus on prolactin as a metabolic hormone. Trends Endocrinol 2006;17:110–116.
41 Vega SA, Hollmann W, Struder HK: Influences of exercise and training on the circulating concentration of prolactin in humans. J Neuroendocrinol 2011;24:395–402.
42 Viru A, Viru M: Biochemical Monitoring of Sport Training. Champaign, Human Kinetics, 2001.
43 Daly W, Seegers CA, Rubin DA, Dobridge JD, Hackney AC: Relationship between stress hormones and testosterone with prolonged endurance exercise. Eur J Appl Physiol 2005;93:375–380.
44 Radomski MW, Cross M, Buguet A: Exercise-induced hyperthermia and hormonal responses to exercise. Can J Physiol Pharmacol 1998;76:547–552.
45 Hackney AC: Characterization of the prolactin response to prolonged endurance exercise. Acta Kinesiol Univ Tartu 2008;13:31–38.
46 Ansley L, Marvin G, Sharma A, Kendall MJ, Jones DA, Bridge MW: The effects of head cooling on endurance and neuroendocrine responses to exercise in warm conditions. Physiol Res 2008;57:863–872.
47 Hackney AC, Ness RJ, Schreiber A: Effects of endurance exercise on nocturnal hormone concentrations in males. Chronobiol Int 1989;6:341–346.
48 Hackney AC, Premo MC, McMurray RJ: Influence of aerobic versus anaerobic exercise on the relationship between reproductive hormones in men. J Sports Sci 1995;13:305–311.
49 Hackney AC, Sharp RL, Runyan WS, Ness RJ: Relationship of resting prolactin and testosterone in males during intensive training. Br J Sports Med 1989;23:194.

50 Wheeler GD, Wall SR, Belcastro AN, Cumming DC: Reduced serum testosterone and prolactin levels in male distance runners. JAMA 1984;252:514–516.
51 Hackney AC, Sharp RL, Runyan W, Kim Y, Ness RJ: Effects of intensive training on the prolactin response to submaximal exercise in males. J Iowa Acad Sci 1989;96:52–53.
52 Boyden TW, Pamenter RW, Grosso D, Stanforth P, Rotkis T, Wilmore JH: Prolactin responses, menstrual cycles, and body composition of women runners. J Clin Endocrinol Metab 1982;54:711–714.
53 Hackney AC, Sinning WE, Bruot BC: Hypothalamic-pituitary-testicular axis function in endurance-trained males. Int J Sports Med 1990;11:298–303.
54 Hackney AC, Dobridge JD: Thyroid hormones and the interrelationship of cortisol and prolactin: influence of prolonged, exhaustive exercise. Endokrynol Pol 2009;60:252–257.
55 Ortega E: Neuroendocrine mediators in the modulation of phagocytosis by exercise: physiological implications. Exerc Immunol Rev 2003;9:70–93.
56 Joyner M, Coyle EF: Endurance exercise performance: the physiology of champions. J Physiol 2008; 586:35–44.

Anthony C. Hackney, PhD, DSc
UNC-CH Fetzer Building – CB 8700
Chapel Hill, NC 27599-8700 (USA)
E-Mail ach@email.unc.edu

Lanfranco F, Strasburger CJ (eds): Sports Endocrinology.
Front Horm Res. Basel, Karger, 2016, vol 47, pp 12–26 (DOI: 10.1159/000445149)

Exercise and the Hypothalamo-Pituitary-Adrenal Axis

Martine Duclos[a–c] · Antoine Tabarin[d]

[a]Department of Sport Medicine and Functional Explorations, G. Montpied Hospital, CHU, [b]INRA, UMR 1019, UNH, Centre de Recherche en Nutrition Humaine d'Auvergne, and [c]Unité de Nutrition Humaine, Clermont Université/Université d'Auvergne, Clermont-Ferrand, and [d]Department of Endocrinology, Hôpital de Haut-Lévêque, CHU de Bordeaux, Pessac, France

Abstract

Exercise represents a potent physiological stimulus upon the hypothalamo-pituitary adrenal (HPA) axis. Two major factors modulate the HPA axis response to exercise: intensity and duration. Endurance training per se does not induce permanent hypercortisolism as endurance-trained subjects have similar biological markers of HPA axis activity in resting condition as healthy untrained men. However, during a challenge of the HPA axis, endurance-trained subjects demonstrate an adaptation of the HPA axis activity to repeated exercise resulting from decreased tissular sensitivity to glucocorticoids. A great diversity of other mechanisms is involved in this adaptation, acting potentially at all levels in the cascade and leading to the biological effects of cortisol.

The activation of the hypothalamo-pituitary-adrenal (HPA) axis represents a physiological response to the energetic, metabolic, vascular, neurophysiological, or psychological needs of exercise. Glucocorticoids (GCs), the end product of the HPA axis, exert many beneficial actions in exercising humans. GCs increase the availability of metabolic substrates for the energy need of muscles, and maintain normal vascular integrity and responsiveness during exercise. In addition, GCs prevent the organism from an overreaction of the immune system in the face of repeated exercise-induced muscle damage [1]. Exercise-trained healthy subjects, which represent physiological models of exercise-induced repeated activation of the HPA axis, show functional integrity of their HPA axis, demonstrating the fine-tuning homeostasis of the HPA axis.

Activation of the Hypothalamic-Pituitary-Adrenal Axis during an Acute Bout of Exercise

During exercise, the HPA axis responds to numerous stimuli reflecting the regulatory and integrative functions of the HPA axis: neuronal homeostatic signals (chemoreceptor, baroreceptor, and osmoreceptor stimulation), circulating homeostatic signals (glucose, leptin, ghrelin, and atrial natriuretic peptide), and inflammatory signals (IL-1, IL-6, and TNF-α) [1].

To gain insight into the brain activation in response to exercise, Timofeeva et al. [2] have realized a full analysis of rat brain regions activated by 90 min of treadmill running. After a session of treadmill running, almost all paraventricular corticotropin-releasing factor neurons express the immediate early gene *c-fos*, a marker of persistent neuronal activity, demonstrating that treadmill running strongly activates the hypophysiotropic corticotropin-releasing hormone (CRH) system. Finally, *c-fos* mRNA expression returned to control levels after a 2-hour recovery.

In humans, repeated brachial blood samplings showed that the dynamics of the HPA axis activation during exercise are associated with the stimulation of hypothalamic CRH and arginine-vasopressin secretion (with a prominent role of CRH), and the synthesis and release of adrenocorticotropic hormone (ACTH) from pituitary corticotropic cells preceding the increase in cortisol [3].

Response to Endurance Exercise

Two major factors modulate the HPA axis response to endurance exercise: *intensity* and *duration* [3, 4]. The minimum intensity of exercise (i.e. threshold) necessary to produce a cortisol response from the HPA axis is 60% of VO_{2max}; thereafter, for exercises above 60% VO_{2max}, plasma cortisol concentrations increase linearly with exercise intensity [5, 6]. Below this intensity threshold, i.e. during light, prolonged exercise (<60% VO_{2max}), ACTH and cortisol concentrations may increase, with a duration threshold of around 90 min of exercise at 40% VO_{2max} [5]. These thresholds are independent of training. Indeed, when exercise is realized at similar relative intensity (%VO_{2max}) between untrained and trained men, the thresholds of intensity and duration for exercise-induced cortisol secretion are similar between the two groups as well as the magnitude and duration of cortisol increases [5, 7–9].

Other factors can modulate the cortisol response to exercise: *hypohydration*, *meals*, and *time of day*. Independently of external thermal stress, hypohydration (up to 4.8% body mass loss) potently amplifies the exercise-induced responses of cortisol to exercise. This enhancement of exercise-induced stress probably results from an increased core temperature and cardiovascular demand due to decreased plasma volume [10]. Meals also stimulate cortisol release in humans. Exercise performed immediately after food ingestion results in a blunted cortisol response to the exercise stimulus, and, conversely, the postprandial increase in serum cortisol concentrations is attenuated by prior exercise [11]. Finally, as the cortisol response to exercise is significantly modulated by time of day, which influences the incremental response (greater increase in the evening than in the morning), but not the peak response to exercise, neglecting the circadian cortisol variations may introduce bias in the interpretation of hormone responses to exercise and training [12, 13]. To investigate whether circadian and diurnal rhythms underlying the secretion of cortisol modulate the HPA axis response to aerobic exercise, Kanaley et al. [12] submitted moderately trained male subjects to 30 min of treadmill running at ~85% VO_{2max}. The cortisol response to exercise was significantly modulated by time of day: although the duration of the increase in serum cortisol concentrations after exercise was similar (150–155 min) at 07.00, 19.00, and 24.00 h, the increase over control day levels was greatest at 24.00 h and smallest at 19.00 h; an intermediate response occurred at 07.00 h, with a rebound suppression of cortisol release for about 50 min after exercise at 24.00 h but not 07.00 or 19.00 h. These differences in serum cortisol concentrations between exercise and control days were transient (~40–130 min) and were most apparent when effects over time were studied, as the 6-hour integrated cortisol concentrations (1 h before and 5 h after the start of exercise) did not differ significantly at each time of day. The strengths of this study were (1) the control for possible effects of meals (standard last meal 12 h before exercise), sleep (no sleep during the 5-hour period following the start of exercise), and prior exercise, and (2) the comparison of the pattern of cortisol release over time under exercise conditions with that observed at rest at the identical time of day for each subject. Early studies did not include a control day and simply compared cortisol concentrations during exercise to levels before exercise on the same day. Altogether, these results reinforce those of Thuma et al. [13] and demonstrate that it is mandatory to consider the clock dependence of the HPA axis to interpret the cortisol responses to exercise and training.

When repeated daily bouts of exercise are performed, the *recovery time between the sessions* may also influence the HPA response to following bouts of exercise. In male elite endurance athletes, the repetition of a prolonged strenuous exercise (bout of 75 min of exercise at 75% VO_{2max}) induces a more pronounced increase in ACTH and cortisol when the previous bout of exercise was performed 3 h as compared to 6 h earlier. This enhancement of the HPA axis activity during repetition of exercise occurs despite completely normalized plasma concentrations of cortisol and ACTH between the two exercise sessions. These data support the hypothesis that the duration of rest between the first and the second exercise is a significant determinant for the magnitude of the cortisol response during reactivation of the HPA axis by the second bout of exercise [14]. Finally, as cortisol also prepares the organism for the next bout of exercise (consolidating glycogen reserve in muscle tissue and shutting off muscle inflammatory reactions) [1], when an acute bout of intensive or prolonged exercise is stopped, cortisol levels may return to pre-exercise values with a delay. This delay does not exceed more than 150 min after the end of exercise [3].

Response to Resistance Exercise

Resistance (strength) exercise is also a potent stimulus to the HPA axis. In humans, a bout of resistance exercise acutely increased cortisol secretion and then plasma cortisol concentrations [15].

Two major factors modulate the HPA axis response to resistance exercise: the intensity and the volume (sets × repetitions × intensity) of the exercise performed. Resistance protocols, moderate to high in intensity, high in volume, stressing large muscle mass and using short rest intervals produce the greatest acute hormonal elevations (ACTH and cortisol) [15].

The role of cortisol during resistance exercise is multiple: meeting the greater metabolic demand of resistance training, remodeling of muscles in response to a bout of exercise as cortisol regulates muscle protein content by inhibiting muscle protein synthesis, and stimulating protein degradation likely via activation of the ubiquitin pathway. In addition to these well-known effects, cortisol can also influence neuromuscular function (i.e. neuronal activity, intracellular signaling, and muscle force) through various rapid or short-term mechanisms [16]. Cortisol may contribute to the muscular properties of the peripheral nervous system by rapidly modulating Ca^{2+} influx in skeletal muscle cells [16].

The type of muscle contraction may also modulate HPA axis responses to resistance exercise. Lifting a weight during dynamic resistance exercise necessitates force production during muscle shortening (concentric contraction) whereas lowering a weight (eccentric contraction) requires force production during muscle lengthening. Resistance training is usually performed with concentric and eccentric contractions at the same constant load. Eccentric training presents several advantages at similar muscle load [for a review see 17]: during resistance exercise, the effects of gravity, and mechanical properties of the sarcomere and connective tissue in skeletal muscle allow a greater muscle load during an eccentric (lengthening) muscle contraction than a concentric (shortening) muscle contraction. Thus, some evidence suggests that, at similar muscle load, cortisol levels will increase less over time with concentric muscle actions compared to eccentric muscle actions [15].

Adaptation of the Hypothalamic-Pituitary-Adrenal Axis to Exercise Training

Normal Functional Activity of the Hypothalamic-Pituitary-Adrenal Axis in Trained Subjects

Since the last decade, evidence accumulates showing that in endurance-trained subjects, 24-hour cortisol secretion *is not* increased under nonexercising conditions. Accordingly, plasma cortisol at 08.00 h, nycthemeral cortisol rhythm, overnight and 24-hour urinary free cortisol (UFC), seasonal rhythmicity of cortisol excretion, and cortisol response to the dexamethasone suppression test in resting endurance-trained subjects are similar to those of age-matched untrained subjects [5, 9, 12, 18].

Moreover, endurance-trained subjects maintained the seasonal rhythmicity of cortisol excretion. In untrained men, highest concentrations of urinary cortisol, morning plasma cortisol and saliva cortisol are observed during winter and fall compared with spring and summer [3]. In endurance-trained men, such seasonal variations in cortisol secretion have been reported in triathletes and elite cyclists [3, 9].

It should be pointed out that overnight UFC is also similar between endurance-trained subjects and untrained subjects [9]. A reason for pointing out these data is that the sleeping time represents the period where the hormonal profile is the most anabolic [increased ratio of growth hormone (GH) to cortisol and of testosterone to cortisol] [18], and, therefore, the most favorable phase to exercise recovery and protein synthesis. Moreover, activation of the HPA axis during the night results in more severe metabolic consequences than during the day. In this perspective, it has been shown that a physiological increase in plasma cortisol levels in the evening has more pronounced deleterious effects on glucose regulation than elevation of cortisol levels in the morning [19].

Altogether, these results probe the functional integrity of the HPA axis in endurance-trained subjects. The overactivity of the HPA axis reported by some authors [6] may represent a further step in the intensity of the physical activity strain, leading to overreaching and/or overtraining, and pathological adaptations of the HPA axis. As suggested by Luger et al. [6], the highly trained people that they studied and who presented with mild evening hypercortisolism may have included subjects whose personalities had anorectic or depressive components, all conditions associated with chronic activation of the HPA axis. In women, alterations in the HPA axis in amenorrheic runners have been reported, with UFC levels elevated to levels observed in anorexia nervosa. However, the pathophysiology of this increased cortisol secretion has been extensively explained by De Souza et al. [20] and Loucks and Thuma [21] who repeatedly demonstrated that it is the stress of chronic energy deficiency (negative energy balance) which induces hypercortisolism and not the stress of exercise by itself which induces this chronic hypercortisolism.

Temporary Exercise-Induced Cortisol Secretion and Balanced 24-Hour Cortisol Secretion in Endurance-Trained Subjects

Exercise of sufficient intensity and/or duration increases cortisol secretion. However, whatever the type and the duration of exercise, in nonovertrained subjects, the exercise-induced cortisol increase does not exceed more than 120–150 min after the end of exercise [5, 7, 8, 12, 18, 21, 22]. This raises the following question: is there a decrease in cortisol production after these 2 h of exercise recovery that could explain the finding of similar average 24-hour cortisol concentrations between exercising and nonexercising subjects? Unfortunately, data are lacking to answer accurately to this question.

In a study conducted by Kern et al. [18], 10 trained healthy men participated in a balanced crossover study including three conditions: (1) no exercise, (2) long-duration exercise of low intensity (biking 40 km from 18.00 to 20.30 h), and (3) long-duration exercise of moderate intensity (biking 120–150 km from 16.00 to 20.30 h). During the subsequent night, somnopolygraphic sleep recordings were obtained and blood was collected every 15 min for the determination of plasma concentrations of cortisol. At the end of long-duration exercise of low intensity, plasma cortisol levels did not significantly differ from the baseline value before exercise (400 nmol/l) whereas cortisol was significantly elevated at the end of the long-duration exercise of moderate intensity (1,000 nmol/l). During the no-exercise night, the typical secretory cortisol patterns were present with nadir cortisol concentrations during the first half of sleep but increased cortisol levels during the second part of sleep. Average concentrations of cortisol during the nights did not depend on whether this night was preceded by a period of exercise or not. Separate analysis of the first and second parts of the night indicated that, in the long-duration exercise of moderate intensity, cortisol levels were increased during the first half of the night whereas the rise in cortisol concentrations during the second half of the night was reduced. Therefore, average cortisol concentrations at night remained unaffected between no exercise and exercise days. Hackney and Viru [23] also reported that cortisol is suppressed at night after daytime exercise involving two bouts of moderate-intensity exercise (aerobic) or high-intensity exercise (anaerobic). However, in the control condition of this study (no exercise), plasma cortisol levels during the first part of the night (between 22.00 and 02.00 h) averaged at 250 nmol/l. These concentrations are increased compared to the expected value in sleeping subjects, a finding that suggests that the postexercise-induced decrease in cortisol at night may have been underestimated.

Nindl et al. [22] monitored hormone levels in young healthy men during the night following an acute heavy-resistance exercise performed in the late afternoon (from 15.00 to 17.00 h). The protocol of exercise was designed to be a high-volume workout (i.e. high total work) that recruited and activated a large amount of muscle tissue. This was accomplished by performing multijoint exercises that required the use of major muscle groups in the lower and upper body. After the completion of the last set, blood was sampled every 10 min from 17.00 to 18.00 h and thereafter every hour until 06.00 h on the following morning. Compared to a control day without any exercise, cortisol levels were significantly increased at the end of exercise (7.1 vs. 16.9 μg/dl, control vs. exercise trial), remained elevated 2 h after the end of exercise, and restored to control (resting) values thereafter, but were not lower than the day without exercise. Therefore, the influence of resistance exercise on cortisol concentration does not appear to be long lasting, neither does it suppress significantly nighttime cortisol secretion. But, once again, it remains difficult to conclude definitely on the effects of exercise on 24-hour cortisol secretion as the sleep patterns have not been evaluated in this study.

Compared with repeated plasma sampling, 24-hour UFC is less invasive and allows normal and usual conditions of life. We have shown that in swimmers during a training and/or a competition day, 24-hour UFC excretion, a testimony of 24-hour cortisol secretion, remained within the normal range of the laboratory [24]. Moreover, in comparison with untrained men [unpubl. results], endurance-trained men presented similar 24-hour UFC than untrained men. These findings are in agreement with the finding of similar 24-hour UFC levels between the 2 hard training days and the 2 rest days in eumenorrheic women running more than 92.5 km per week for the past 12 months, or between the 2 hard training days and the 2 rest days in the eumenorrheic runners and the 2 rest days in eumenorrheic untrained women.

As the nocturnal period is essential for exercise recovery, Gouarne et al. [9] have studied the overnight GC output to assess the delicate balance between cumulative fatigue resulting from exercise training and its recovery period over a 10-month season in triathletes. In endurance-trained men and untrained men, overnight urinary cortisol excretion showed seasonal variations, whereas the urinary cortisol/cortisone ratio remained stable with no training effect. This also suggests that any increase in cortisol secretion may be balanced by its parallel inactivation into cortisone. In women, compared to their untrained peers, Boisseau et al. [25] showed no training effect on resting urinary excretion of cortisol, cortisone and the cortisol/cortisone ratio.

Contrary to their apparently similar resting HPA axis activity, endurance-trained subjects differ from untrained subjects when their HPA axis is challenged.

Endurance Training and Response to Mild Stress

In both women [26] and men [27], regular physical exercise leads to reduced stress reactivity and improved stress recovery from psychosocial stress when compared to physically inactive subjects. In these studies, stress was induced by a standardized and validated psychosocial stressor. Interestingly, in the study of Klaperski et al. [26], this effect is observed both in the highly active (7–12 h/week) and in the moderately active groups (2–6 h/week) showing that this is not restricted to highly trained athletes. Moreover, in women studied during the luteal phase where free salivary cortisol reactivity reached its maximum, response was comparable to the male response [27].

Endurance Training and Response to Strong Physical and Physiological Stimuli

Differences between endurance-trained subjects and untrained subjects are also obvious when HPA axis testing is performed during the immediate postexercise recovery, a time when cortisol is still increased by the preceding bout of exercise (fig. 1a). These differences can be summarized as follows: when HPA testing is conducted after exercise-induced increases in plasma cortisol concentrations, the ability of the HPA axis of trained subjects to respond to a second physiological challenge (food intake [5] or exercise [5, 14]) or to a pharmacological challenge (ACTH 250 μg or corticotropin-releasing factor/lysine vasopressine test [28]) is not impaired. On the contrary, this ability to respond to a second stimulation, in face of exercise-induced cortisol, is lost in untrained subjects. These results suggest decreased pituitary sensitivity to the early GC negative feedback in endurance-trained athletes. The cortisol response to food intake also illustrates this difference. In untrained men, Brandenberger et al. [11] showed that the daily cortisol pattern results from the interactions between the meal-related peaks,

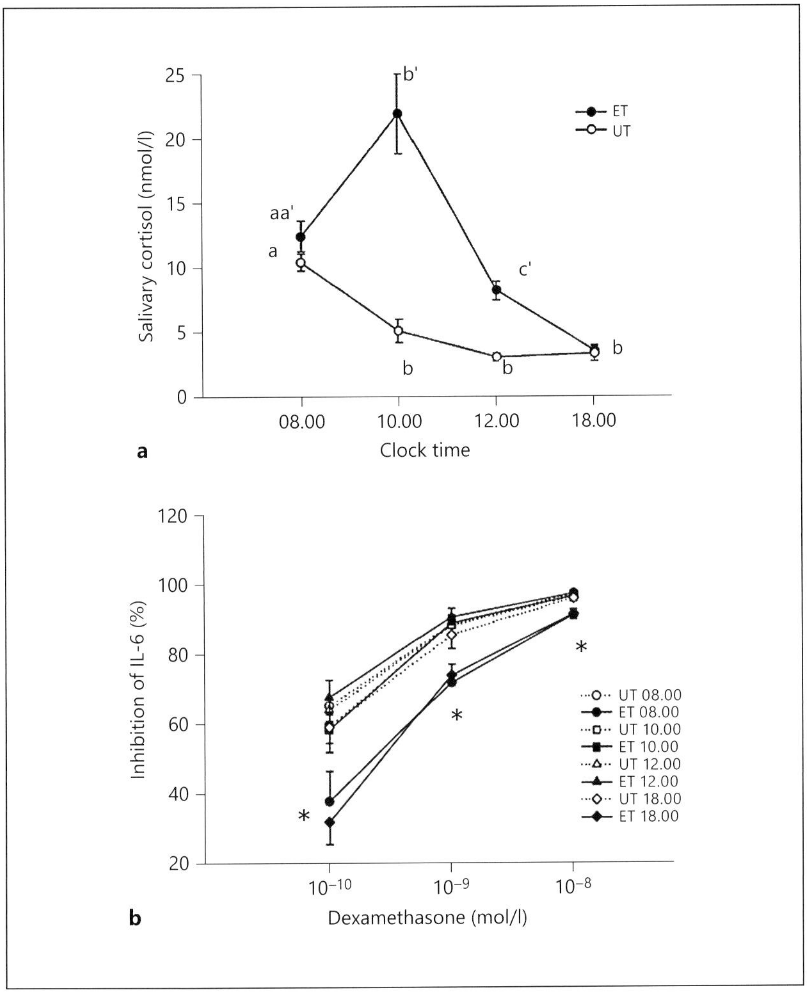

Fig. 1. a Salivary cortisol concentrations across time during the experimental day in endurance-trained men (ET; exercise and resting sessions) and untrained men (UT; resting session). ET men realized a 2-hour run between 08.00 and 10.00 h. Bars not sharing a common letter are significantly different from each other. Results are means ± SEM [8]. At 08.00 h, salivary cortisol concentrations were similar between UT and ET men; 2 h of exercise induced an increase in cortisol at the end of exercise (10.00 h) and 2 h after the end of exercise (12.00 h; ET). **b** Percentage inhibition of lipopolysaccharide (0.3 µg/ml)-stimulated IL-6 production in cultures of peripheral monocytes in ET (solid lines) and UT men (dotted lines). The percent values of dexamethasone-induced IL-6 inhibition are significantly lower in ET at 08.00 and 18.00 h compared with their values at 10.00 and 12.00 h, and compared with the values of UT men at 08.00 h, 10.00, 12.00 and 18.00 h (* $p < 0.05$) [8]. The sensitivity to GC in UT men is similar at every time sampling between 08.00 and 18.00 h despite different plasma cortisol levels (**a**). At 08.00 h, monocytes of ET men were less sensitive to dexamethasone than those of UT men (**b**). An acute exercise (between 08.00 and 10.00 h) increased the sensitivity of monocytes to GC in ET men to the levels assayed in control ET men.

especially the major midday cortisol peak, and the exercise-induced cortisol increases, both of which inhibit the responses to subsequent stimulation. It explains why in conditions of exercise-induced marked cortisol increase, the subsequent stimulation exerted by a meal taken 60 min after a 2-hour run did not elicit a rise in cortisol levels in untrained men [5]. By contrast, endurance-trained men, despite similar increases in cortisol concentrations, are able to escape the blunting effect of the preceding exercise-induced cortisol increase (GC feedback) and, therefore, to respond to subsequent stimulation with a significant cortisol increase to noon meal [5].

Different mechanisms can be involved in these changes. At the level of the central nervous system, neuropeptides and corticosteroid receptors [glucocorticoid (GR) and mineralocorticoid receptors] in the brain and anterior pituitary play a major role in the regulation of circulating cortisol levels. The influence of exercise on these central regulators in humans is largely unexplored for evident methodological reasons. In animals, studies investigating the mechanisms underlying the potential influences of exercise training on the central regulation of HPA axis activity and reactivity have used forced exercise protocols (treadmill training or swimming). In rats and mice, forced exercise induces different regulatory changes in the HPA axis compared to voluntary exercise and must be regarded as a chronic stress paradigm. Using voluntary access to a running wheel, long-term (4-week) exercising mice, after a transiently elevated activity of the HPA axis, normalize the 24-hour activity of the HPA axis [29, 30]. This restoration in HPA axis activity in healthy rats resulted from adaptations in the hypothalamus and adrenal gland that promote a lower CRH production and reduced adrenal sensitivity to ACTH, respectively [29, 30]. Moreover, similar changes in HPA axis responses than those reported in humans were observed after subjecting long-term (4-week) exercised animals to a stressful challenge. Exercised rats or mice show lower GC responses than control, untrained animals when exposed to a novel environment [29]. As commented by Droste et al. [29]:

> This seems to reflect the exercised animals' decreased anxiety-related behavior observed in the novel cage and in specific anxiety tests. However, if animals are confronted with the stronger psychological and physical stimulus of forced swimming then the exercised animals, as compared to the controls, respond with higher glucocorticoid levels. Given that the forced swim situation is a potentially life-threatening situation and involves increased metabolic demand, the enhanced hormone response is considered to be a better adaptive response. The exercised animals also showed stronger (glucocorticoid-dependent) memory formation of the event. Thus, exercise benefits appropriate glucocorticoid response to stressful events.

At the peripheral level, tissular sensitivity to GC can also be different in endurance-trained subjects. The response to GCs is regulated not only by the GC concentration but also by the availability of cortisol and the GC sensitivity of the target tissues. Changes in GC availability and/or sensitivity may explain the apparent discrepancy between repeated and prolonged exercise-induced HPA axis activation (during exercise and 1–2 h after exercise) and the lack of metabolic consequences of such increased cortisol secretion. Duclos et al. [8] have reported an in vitro plasticity of monocyte sensitivity to GC in endurance-trained men, superimposed on changes in systemic cortisol concentrations. Compared to untrained men, and despite similar resting cortisol levels, the sensitivity of monocytes to GC in endurance-trained men is decreased 8 and 24 h after the end of the last training session (fig. 1b). Moreover, in these endurance-trained subjects, an acute bout of exercise increased the sensitivity of monocytes to GC to the levels assayed in untrained men (fig. 1b). This decreased sensitivity of monocytes to GC in endurance-trained men 24 h after the last bout of exercise may be related to a process of desensitization supposed to protect the body from the long-lasting exercise-induced cortisol secretion. However, this variation in tissular sensitivity (immune system) to GC cannot not be generalized to all body tissues owing to the well-known variability in GC sensitivity across the immune and the cardiovascular system, and the HPA axis within healthy subjects [31].

Upstream these intracellular mechanisms, the extra- and/or the intracellular cortisol availability could also be modified. Extracellular bioavailability depends on the free fraction of cortisol. Cortisol largely binds to plasma proteins and especially to the cortisol-binding globulin (CBG). Thus plasma cortisol levels are modulated by variations in CBG and poorly correlate with cortisol production rates unless differences in CBG are corrected [4]. Salivary cortisol concentrations closely reflect the free – active – plasma cortisol [4]. Measuring simultaneously plasma and saliva cortisol concentrations, we did not find differences in endurance-trained men versus untrained men during resting conditions as well as exercise [7, 8, 32]. In addition to CBG which modulates the extracellular availability of cortisol, another level of control of the effect of cortisol on target cells is exerted by the prereceptor metabolism of cortisol by the tissue-specific enzyme 11β-hydroxysteroid dehydrogenase (11β-HSD) which interconverts hormonally active cortisol and inactive cortisone, and has been shown to modulate cortisol hormone action in several peripheral tissue [33]. The crucial physiological principle illuminated by the action of 11β-HSD is that cortisol action on target cells is determined by enzyme activity within the cells rather than by circulating cortisol levels alone. Using this approach, the 24-hour urinary cortisol/cortisone ratio (an index of whole-body 11β-HSD activity) was reported to be negatively related to the total training load in a population of swimmers [27]. This suggests that any significant increase in 24-hour cortisol secretion is counterbalanced by its parallel inactivation into cortisone. The nocturnal period is essential for exercise recovery. Gouarne et al. [9] have studied the overnight GC output to assess the delicate balance between cumulative fatigue resulting from exercise training and its recovery period over a 10-month season in triathletes. To dissociate the effects of training from those of seasonal hormonal variations, endurance-trained men were compared to untrained men. Gouarne et al. [9] reported similar overnight urinary cortisol output in both groups during the 10-month follow-up. Moreover, whereas overnight urinary cortisol excretion showed seasonal variations (November > June) in both groups, conversely urinary cortisol/cortisone excretion remained stable in both groups during the follow-up period, suggesting again that any significant increase in cortisol secretion (seasonal-induced increased cortisol secretion) is counterbalanced by its parallel inactivation of cortisone. The importance of this mechanism is also suggested by the observation of 2 triathletes who developed an overtraining syndrome (decreased performance, high score of fatigue, and inability of maintaining the training load) during the follow-up: these subjects presented a sharp decrease in the inactivation of cortisol into cortisone with an increased cortisol/cortisone ratio compared to their basal level (values before training) and compared to the values of the other triathletes at the same period.

Finally, exercise training could lead to a modulation of GR expression.

Animal research using the stress of a treadmill running – and not voluntary wheel running – has identified a reduction in GR content (in renal, myocardial, and hepatic cytosol) after an endurance exercise bout with endurance training also reducing GR content in an intensity- and load-volume-dependent manner [34]. Evidence from cross-sectional studies in humans supports the results in peripheral blood mononuclear cells (GR mRNA), both in response to an acute exercise session and training [35]. However, whether or not the immune cell GRs exhibit similar patterns of change with exercise and training than muscle, adipose tissue and/or central GRs remains highly speculative in humans.

Other Modulators of Hypothalamic-Pituitary-Adrenal Axis Responsiveness to Exercise Training

Most of the studies mentioned above focused on the effects of exercise and training on the HPA axis using plasma cortisol concentrations. However, cortisol concentrations result from a dynamic process including secretion and clearance. Other important endocrine features include transport proteins, hormone-protein dissociation, hormone degradation rates, and the intra- and paracrine pathways. The physiological meaning of the free and total cortisol adds to this complexity, as outlined in the above paragraphs. The responses may also depend upon the actions and interactions of other hormone steroid metabolites, neurotransmitters, peptides, amines, and growth factors.

In response to an acute resistance exercise session, various circulating hormone concentrations increase (cortisol, GH, adrenaline, noradrenaline, and testosterone). In response to an acute endurance exercise session, mainly circulating concentrations of cortisol and GH increase, whereas in case of prolonged exercise (90 min) testosterone decreased in men [4–6].

Role of Estradiol and Gender

Most studies examining the follicular and luteal phases reported no effect of the menstrual cycle phase on the basal activity and responses of the HPA axis to exercise (whatever the type and the intensity of exercise) [25]. Exercises of high and moderate intensity (90 and 70% VO_{2max}) did not elicit any difference in plasma ACTH and cortisol responses to exercise during the follicular and the luteal phase of the menstrual cycle. Similar conclusions were drawn following endurance exercise (75% maximum heart rate) or resistance exercise sessions in cross-trained women [25].

However, as CBG varies in healthy eumenorrheic women during the menstrual cycle [36], it is important to measure cortisol availability in relation with exercise. Only Kirschbaum et al. [36] and our team [25] have investigated the response of free cortisol surrogates instead of plasma cortisol: salivary cortisol [25, 36] and urinary cortisol [25]. All authors reported a lack of differences in salivary cortisol responses between the early follicular and the luteal phase in eumenorrheic untrained and trained women at rest and in response to endurance exercise (limited-time exercise: 30–40 min at 75% VO_{2max}).

Altogether, these studies suggest that physiological variations in endogenous sex steroids during the menstrual cycle have no effect on HPA axis activity and reactivity to exercise stimulation, whether total plasma cortisol [6–8, 24, 25] or its free fraction is considered, both in salivary and in urinary samples [25]. Notably, these results extended to peripheral metabolism of cortisol with no difference in urinary free cortisone excretion across the menstrual cycle at rest and in response to exercise [25].

Effect of Oral Contraceptives

It is well documented that ethinyl estradiol contained in oral contraceptive (OC) pills increases CBG hepatic production, increasing serum cortisol-binding capacity and total cortisol concentration [36].

Surprisingly, although the use of OC is increasing worldwide and this at younger age, few studies have investigated HPA axis activity and reactivity in women using OC. To the best of our knowledge, only four studies have examined the association between OC use and free cortisol, showing a blunted salivary free cortisol response to physical, psychological stress or ACTH stimulation, suggesting that higher CBG levels may lead to lower salivary free cortisol responses to stress [25]. Such an investigation is of major importance as relative hypocortisolemia may have multiple clinical/health consequences (chronic fatigue syndrome, fibromyalgia, and burnout.

Our team investigated trained and untrained women, OC users and non-OC users (tested in the follicular and the luteal phase) at rest and during exercise, and showed that whereas estradiol fluctuation during the menstrual cycle phase does not change free cortisol values at baseline and in response to exercise, OC use is associated with increased morning free resting salivary concentrations and urinary cortisol excretion with blunted salivary cortisol responses to prolonged exercise stimulation. To our knowledge, only two other studies have dealt with HPA axis responses to exercise in OC users. Bonen et al. [37] reported that total plasma cortisol increased in eumenorrheic women but not in OC users during and after heavy treadmill exercise. Kirschbaum et al. [36] provided evidence for attenuated salivary cortisol responses to an exhaustive exercise test in young OC users (20 µg ≤ ethinyl estradiol ≥50 µg). OC users were able to respond to a short-term exhaustive bicycle test with a significant increase in free cortisol, but with lower amplitude than women in follicular or luteal phases of their menstrual cycle. By contrast, our team reported no exercise-induced increase in cortisol secretion, which fits well with this increased cortisol secretion. Interestingly, this effect was reported later in the day (12.00–14.00 h and 15.00–19.00 h) than in our study and in conditions where salivary cortisol was not increased compared to non-OC users, suggesting other mechanisms explaining this blunted cortisol response to stimulation.

Further studies will be necessary to determine the long-term consequences of these modifications in HPA axis activity and reactivity in women using OC.

Conclusion

Exercise-trained subjects have similar HPA axis activity in resting condition than healthy untrained subjects. However, when the HPA axis is challenged, exercise-trained subjects and mainly endurance-trained subjects demonstrate a decreased pituitary (and probably hypothalamic and/or suprahypothalamic) sensitivity to the negative feedback of GC that explain their capacity to achieve successfully a second bout of exercise separated by a short rest period. Adaptation to exercise-induced repeated and prolonged cortisol secretion also includes decreased peripheral tissue sensitivity to GCs that is supposed to protect the body from the severe metabolic and immune consequences of increased cortisol levels. A great diversity of mechanisms is involved in such adaptation, acting potentially at all levels in the cascade and leading to the biological effects of cortisol. These beneficial effects of regular exercise on the HPA axis are evidenced by stress resilience but also in case of pathological functional hyperactivity of the HPA axis (visceral obesity and metabolic disorders) where physical activity is a cornerstone of management of the disease. Finally, one might wonder if the physically inactive subjects are the best physiological model to study the activity and reactivity of the HPA axis as our genes are programmed to be highly physically active.

References

1 Sapolsky RM, Romero M, Munck AU: How do glucocorticoids influence stress responses? Integrating permissive, suppressive, stimulatory, and preparative actions. Endocr Rev 2000;21:55–89.

2 Timofeeva E, Huang Q, Richard D: Effects of treadmill running on brain activation and the corticotropin-releasing hormone system. Neuroendocrinology 2003;77:388–405.

3 Duclos M, Tabarin A: Exercise, training and the hypothalamo-pituitary-adrenal axis; in Ghigo E, Lanfranco F, Strasburger CJ (eds): Hormone Use and Abuse by Athletes. New York, Springer, 2009, pp 9–16.

4 Duclos M, Guinot M, Le Bouc **Y**: Cortisol and GH: odd and controversial ideas. Appl Physiol Nutr Metab 2007;32:895–903.

5 Duclos M, Corcuff JB, Rashedi M, Fougere V, Manier G: Trained versus untrained men: different immediate post-exercise responses of pituitary-adrenal axis. A preliminary study. Eur J Appl Physiol 1997; 75:343–350.

6 Luger A, Deuster PA, Kyle SB, Gallucci WT, Montgomery LC, Gold PW, Lynn Loriaux D, Chrousos GP: Acute hypothalamic-pituitary-adrenal responses to the stress of treadmill exercise. N Engl J Med 1987;316:1309–1315.

7 Duclos M, Minkhar M, Sarrieau A, Bonnemaison D, Manier G, Mormede P: Reversibility of endurance training-induced changes on glucocorticoid sensitivity of monocytes by an acute exercise. Clin Endocrinol (Oxf) 1999;51:749–756.
8 Duclos M, Gouarne C, Bonnemaison D: Acute and chronic effects of exercise on tissue sensitivity to glucocorticoids. J Appl Physiol (1985) 2003;94:869–875.
9 Gouarne C, Groussard C, Gratas-Delamarche A, Delamarche P, Duclos M: Overnight urinary cortisol and cortisone add new insights into adaptation to training. Med Sci Sports Exerc 2005;37:1157–1167.
10 Judelson DA, Maresh CM, Yamamoto LM, Farrell MJ, Armstrong LE, Kraemer WJ, Volek JS, Spiering BA, Casa DJ, Anderson JM: Effect of hydration state on resistance exercise-induced endocrine markers of anabolism, catabolism, and metabolism. J Appl Physiol (1985) 2008;105:816–824.
11 Brandenberger G, Follenius M, Hietter B, Reinhardt B, Simeoni M: Feedback from meal-related peaks determines diurnal changes in cortisol response to exercise. J Clin Endocrinol Metab 1982;54:592–594.
12 Kanaley JA, Weltman JY, Pieper KS, Weltman A, Hartman ML: Cortisol and growth hormone responses to exercise at different times of day. J Clin Endocrinol Metab 2001;86:2881–2889.
13 Thuma JR, Gilders R, Verdun M, Loucks AB: Circadian rhythm of cortisol confounds cortisol responses to exercise: implications for future research. J Appl Physiol Cell Physiol 1995;78:1657–1664.
14 Ronsen O, Kjeldsen-Kragh J, Haug E, Bahr R, Pedersen BK: Recovery time affects immunoendocrine responses to a second bout of endurance exercise. Am J Physiol 2002;283:C1612–C1620.
15 Kraemer RR, Castracane VD: Endocrine alterations from concentric vs. eccentric muscle actions: a brief review. Metabolism 2015;64:190–201.
16 Crewther BT, Cook C, Cardinale M, Weatherby RP, Lowe T: Two emerging concepts for elite athletes: the short-term effects of testosterone and cortisol on the neuromuscular system and the dose-response training role of these endogenous hormones. Sports Med 2011;41:103–123.
17 Isner-Horobeti ME, Dufour SP, Vautravers P, Geny B, Coudeyre E, Richard R: Eccentric exercise training: modalities, applications and perspectives. Sports Med 2013;43:483–512.
18 Kern W, Perras B, Wodick R, Fehm HL, Born J: Hormonal secretion during nighttime sleep indicating stress of daytime exercise. J Appl Physiol (1985) 1995;79:1461–1468.
19 Plat L, Leproult R, L'Hermite-Baleriaux M, Fery F, Mockel J, Polonsky KS, Van Cauter E: Metabolic effects of short-term elevations of plasma cortisol are more pronounced in the evening than in the morning. J Clin Endocrinol Metab 1999;84:3082–3092.
20 De Souza MJ, Van Heest J, Demers LM, Lasley BL: Luteal phase deficiency in recreational runners: evidence for a hypometabolic state. J Clin Endocrinol Metab 2003;88:337–346.
21 Loucks AB, Thuma JR: Luteinizing hormone pulsatility is disrupted at a threshold of energy availability in regularly menstruating women. J Clin Endocrinol Metab 2003;88:297–311.
22 Nindl BC, Kraemer WJ, Deaver DR, Peters JL, Marx JO, Heckman JT, Loomis GA: LH secretion and testosterone concentrations are blunted after resistance exercise in men. J Appl Physiol (1985) 2001;91:1251–1258.
23 Hackney AC, Viru A: Twenty-four-hour cortisol response to multiple daily exercise sessions of moderate and high intensity. Clin Physiol 1999;19:178–182.
24 Atlaoui D, Duclos M, Gouarne C, Lacoste L, Barale F, Chatard JC: The 24-h urinary cortisol/cortisone ratio for monitoring training in elite swimmers. Med Sci Sports Exerc 2004;36:218–224.
25 Boisseau N, Enea C, Diaz V, Dugue B, Corcuff JB, Duclos M: Oral contraception but not menstrual cycle phase is associated with increased free cortisol levels and low HPA axis reactivity. J Endocrinol Invest 2013;36:955–964.
26 Klaperski S, von Dawans B, Heinrichs M, Fuchs R: Does the level of physical exercise affect physiological and psychological responses to psychological stress in women? Psychol Sport Exerc 2013;14:266–274.
27 Rimmele U, Zellweger BC, Marti B, Seiler R, Mohiyeddini C, Ehlert U, Heinrichs M: Trained men show lower cortisol, heart rate and psychological responses to psychosocial stress compared with untrained men. Psychoneuroendocrinology 2007;32:627–635.
28 Duclos M, Corcuff JB, Pehourcq F, Tabarin A: Decreased pituitary sensitivity to glucocorticoids in endurance trained men. Eur J Endocrinol 2001;144:363–368.
29 Droste SK, Collins A, Lightman SL, Linthorst AC, Reul JM: Distinct, time-dependent effects of voluntary exercise on circadian and ultradian rhythms and stress responses of free corticosterone in the rat hippocampus. Endocrinology 2009;150:4170–4179.
30 Campbell JE, Kiraly MA, Atkinson DJ, D'souza AM, Vranic M, Riddell MC: Regular exercise prevents the development of hyperglucocorticoidemia via adaptations in the brain and adrenal glands in male Zucker diabetic fatty rats. Am J Physiol Regul Integr Comp Physiol 2010;299:R168–R176.
31 Ebrecht M, Buske-Kirschbaum A, Hellammer D, Kern S, Rohleder N, Walker B, Kirschbaum C: Tissue specificity of glucocorticoid sensitivity in healthy adults. J Clin Endocrinol Metab 2000;85:3733–3739.

32 Duclos M, Corcuff JB, Arsac L, Moreau-Gaudry F, Rashedi M, Roger P, Tabarin A, Manier G: Corticotroph axis sensitivity after exercise in endurance-trained athletes. Clin Endocrinol (Oxf) 1998;48:493–501.
33 Seckl JR, Walker BR: Minireview: 11β-hydroxysteroid dehydrogenase type 1 – a tissue specific amplifier of glucocorticoid action. Endocrinology 2001;142:1371–1376.
34 Peijie C, Zicai D, Haowen X, Renbao X: Effects of chronic and acute training on glucocorticoid receptors concentrations in rats. Life Sci 2004;75:1303–1311.
35 Bonifazi M, Mencarelli M, Fedele V, Ceccarelli I, Pecorelli A, Grasso G, Aloisi AM, Muscettola M: Glucocorticoid receptor mRNA expression in peripheral blood mononuclear cells in high trained compared to low trained athletes and untrained subjects. J Endocrinol Invest 2009;32:816–820.
36 Kirschbaum C, Kudielka BM, Gaab J, Schommer NC, Hellhammer DH: Impact of gender, menstrual cycle phase, and oral contraceptives on the activity of the hypothalamus-pituitary-adrenal axis. Psychosom Med 1999;61:154–162.
37 Bonen A, Haynes FW, Graham TE: Substrate and hormonal responses to exercise in women using oral contraceptives. J Appl Physiol (1985) 1991;70:1917–1927.

Martine Duclos
Department of Sport Medicine and Functional Explorations
G. Montpied Hospital, CHU, 58, rue Montalembert
FR–63003 Clermont-Ferrand (France)
E-Mail mduclos@chu-clermontferrand.fr

Effects of Physical Activity and Training on Endocrine Function

Lanfranco F, Strasburger CJ (eds): Sports Endocrinology.
Front Horm Res. Basel, Karger, 2016, vol 47, pp 27–43 (DOI: 10.1159/000445154)

Exercise, Training, and the Hypothalamic-Pituitary-Gonadal Axis in Men and Women

Natalia Cano Sokoloff[a] · Madhusmita Misra[a, b] · Kathryn E. Ackerman[a, c]

[a]Neuroendocrine Unit, Massachusetts General Hospital and Harvard Medical School, [b]Pediatric Endocrine Unit, Massachusetts General Hospital for Children and Harvard Medical School, and [c]Division of Sports Medicine, Boston Children's Hospital, Boston, Mass., USA

Abstract

The hypothalamic-pituitary-gonadal (HPG) axis is essential for adequate responses to exercise and training both acutely and chronically. Both testosterone and estrogen play leading roles in neuromuscular adaptation to exercise in males and females. The purpose of this chapter is to illustrate the physiological and pathological changes that occur in the HPG axis secondary to exercise and training. In males, testosterone increases with acute bouts of exercise, but long-term effects are less clear, with evidence of lower testosterone in endurance athletes. Restricted energy availability may negatively affect hormone levels in male endurance athletes, but data regarding low energy availability and its impact on the HPG axis are limited in male athletes. Conversely, in females there is significant evidence that decreased energy availability inhibits the HPG axis, leading to menstrual irregularities and lower bone density. Hormonal changes secondary to acute bouts of exercise are more challenging to interpret in females due to menstrual variability, which traditionally has not been taken into account in many studies. However, some evidence supports an increase in testosterone and estradiol with acute exercise. More work is needed to elucidate the relationships among energy availability, basal hormonal fluctuations, and exercise, and their collective effects on the HPG axis.

An increase in the number of individuals participating in athletics, greater pressure for performance, and sport specialization at a younger age necessitate an understanding of physiological changes that occur in athletes consequent to physical activity. Normal endocrine function is essential for optimal performance, adaptations to exercise, and maintenance of optimal body composition [1, 2]. Effects of long-term training on the reproductive system in female athletes have been widely studied. However, the literature on the endocrine adaptations of male athletes is less robust. This chapter

will review changes in the hypothalamic-pituitary-gonadal (HPG) axis noted acutely and chronically with exercise in both males and females.

Normal functioning of the HPG axis is essential for the onset and maintenance of reproductive function, in addition to immune and musculoskeletal function. Neurons in the hypothalamus secrete gonadotropin-releasing hormone (GnRH), a 10-amino acid neuropeptide. The majority of GnRH neurons are located in the medial basal hypothalamus, the infundibulum and the periventricular region of the hypothalamus. GnRH is released in pulses that vary in amplitude and frequency. The frequency of GnRH secretion modifies the ratio of luteinizing hormone (LH) to follicle-stimulating hormone (FSH) secretion from gonadotropes of the anterior pituitary. Hormones such as prolactin, corticotropin-releasing hormone, glucocorticoids, leptin, adiponectin, ghrelin, insulin, insulin-like growth factor (IGF)-1 and catecholamines, and neurotransmitters such as opiates, modulate the release of GnRH [3].

GnRH receptors are located in pituitary gonadotropes and vary in number depending on gonadotropic secretory capacity. In females, GnRH receptor number varies depending on the phase of the menstrual cycle and is lower during lactation. Certain physiological frequencies of GnRH pulsatility can up-regulate GnRH receptor production, while continuous exposure to GnRH down-regulates its receptors. The GnRH receptor is suppressed by estradiol, progesterone, LH, and FSH, and it is stimulated by calcium, protein kinase C, and a critical level and duration of elevated estradiol [3].

In females, LH is essential for ovulation, androgen production in theca cells, and maintenance of the corpus luteum. FSH stimulates the conversion of androgens to estradiol in granulosa cells and stimulates folliculogenesis. In males, FSH stimulates Sertoli cells to promote spermatogenesis, and LH stimulates Leydig cells to produce testosterone [3].

This chapter will summarize what is known about the short- and long-term effects of training on the reproductive system, focusing on GnRH, gonadotropes, and estradiol and androgen levels, in addition to effects on gametes.

Males

Testosterone

Testosterone is an essential hormone in male athletes both during puberty and adulthood. Changes in androgen levels are of concern because they play an important role in neuromuscular adaptation, muscle maintenance, strength, and aggressiveness in competition [2, 4]. At a cellular level, motor neurons react to testosterone by increasing soma size, dendritic length and synaptic input, and muscle cells respond to testosterone by increasing calcium channels [5]. When given exogenous testosterone, males had an increase in muscle size and/or in performance, both of which increased further if combined with resistance training [6–12].

It has been widely reported that physical activity acutely increases total and free testosterone in men [2, 4, 13]. However, studies of the mid- and long-term effects of exercise on testosterone levels are less clear. Testosterone levels have been shown to be dependent on the time and duration of exercise. Grandys et al. [14] found an increase in serum testosterone after 5 weeks of endurance training on a cycle ergometer in previously untrained healthy men. In a cross-sectional study by Fitzgerald et al. [15], trained cyclists (cycled ≥8 h/week) had higher levels of serum total testosterone compared to recreational athletes (≤30 min of exercise most days of the week). In contrast, multiple cross-sectional studies have found either no difference or a decrease in testosterone in trained endurance athletes compared to controls [16–18]. In a small cross-sectional study that compared runners, cyclists, and elite triathletes against controls, there were no significant differences in FSH, LH, and total or free testosterone levels across groups, but there was a *positive* correlation of training volume and testosterone levels [17]. In a prospective study of cyclists, there were no differences in FSH, LH, or testosterone levels before and after a 300-km bike ride [18].

Multiple cross-sectional studies have found lower testosterone levels in endurance athletes [19–23], resistance-trained athletes [23], soccer players [24], and amateur road cyclists [25] compared to controls. In a prospective study evaluating 14 body builders, half the subjects were required to restrict energy in preparation for competition and half continued to train regularly, but were not allowed to restrict energy to achieve competition weight. Testosterone levels were measured at baseline, 10 and 6 weeks, and 4 days (3 days prior to competition). In the energy-restricted group, testosterone levels were significantly lower at the second two time points versus baseline. In the non-energy-restricted group of body builders, testosterone levels were not significantly different at the beginning and end of the study, but there was a slight decrease in testosterone at the 6-week measurement [26]. Similar to this, Grandys et al. [27] found that testosterone levels vary significantly in sprinters along the annual training period, with testosterone levels higher during low-intensity training and lower during high-intensity training.

Effects of exercise training on testosterone levels may also differ according to age. For example, adult males, but not adolescent boys, were found to have increases in testosterone levels with short bouts of resistance training [28–30]. In a small study of young weight lifters, those who had trained for more than 2 years showed an acute increase in testosterone after resistance exercise, while chronologically age-matched weight lifters who were newer to the sport did not have a significant change [31]. Cross-sectional studies evaluating young gymnasts, soccer players, and hockey players versus age-matched controls did not find differences in testosterone levels among the groups [32, 33]. Prospective studies evaluating changes in testosterone levels in pubertal male athletes are needed.

Addressing the other end of the age spectrum, Häkkinen et al. [34] compared middle-aged (mean age 42 years) and elderly males (mean age 72 years) during 6 months of resistance training and did not find changes in basal free or total testosterone levels

from the beginning to the end of the study, but did find lower basal free testosterone in the older versus younger males. Additionally, they noted comparable acute increases in free and total testosterone after short bouts of exercise both at the beginning and the end of the study in both age groups. Di Luigi et al. [35] showed a high prevalence of low testosterone levels in exercising men above 50 years of age, which raises the concern of undiagnosed hypogonadism in elderly males.

While transient changes in hormone levels after bouts of exercise are notable, effects of different types of habitual exercise on overall testosterone levels may have more clinical utility. There is significant variability in basal testosterone levels and overall hormonal profiles among different sports [36]. It is important to note that hormonal changes involved in overtraining and/or decreased energy availability can decrease the production of testosterone. The overtraining syndrome is defined as the combination of excessive overload with inadequate recovery periods that can result in fatigue and decrease in performance [37]. Currently, no ideal biomarker exists to diagnose overtraining, and despite the somewhat frequent use of a testosterone/cortisol ratio, this potential marker has been found to be unreliable [37]. Hackney et al. [22] showed that highly trained or overtrained male athletes had 40–80% lower levels of testosterone compared to controls.

Safarinejad et al. [38] conducted a well-designed, randomized clinical study of the effects of intensive training versus moderate training in males aged 20–40 years. The high-intensity group (n = 143) performed at approximately 80% of their maximal oxygen uptake (VO_{2max}) while the moderate-intensity group (n = 143) performed at approximately 60% VO_{2max}. Both groups exercised for 2-hour sessions, 5 times a week, for 60 weeks. This was followed by 36 weeks of low-intensity exercise deemed a recovery period. In both groups of exercisers, 60 weeks of exercise resulted in lower free testosterone, FSH, and LH, and higher sex hormone binding globulin (SHBG) and prolactin, with these differences even more pronounced in the high-intensity group. The number of hours of high-intensity exercise significantly correlated negatively with all of the above hormone levels. Moreover, after the administration of exogenous GnRH at the end of the 60 weeks of exercise, both groups had a blunted response of LH and FSH. However, after the recovery phase of 36 weeks of low-intensity exercise, all the parameters returned to normal [38]. This suggests a suppression of the HPG axis, which could be due to a decrease in GnRH production and a reduced response of LH and FSH during habitual exercise.

Leanness and Relative Energy Deficiency in Sport

Participation in sports where leanness is considered a competitive advantage, such as running, cycling, wrestling, lightweight rowing and gymnastics, has been linked to a lower body mass index (BMI) [39], eating disorders [40], and low energy availability [41]. Low energy availability in the context of anorexia nervosa has been associated with low testosterone levels in males [42]. Hagmar et al. [1] evaluated athletes from 26 different sports and divided them into those who participated in leanness sports

and those who did not. The leanness sport athletes had lower body fat, higher spinal bone mineral density (BMD), lower serum free testosterone and leptin, and higher IGF-1 binding protein. The authors suggested that the increase in BMD could be because of the increase in mechanical loading in the specific leanness sports, which presumably overcame the effects of lower testosterone and leptin, both of which are bone anabolic hormones.

In female athletes, low energy availability is a component of the female athlete triad (Triad), a term used to describe the interrelationship of decreased energy availability, subsequent HPG inhibition leading to menstrual irregularity, and decreased BMD [41]. Triad was first described by the American College of Sports Medicine in the 1990s. The International Olympic Committee (IOC) has proposed an expansion of the concept of Triad to include males and has coined the term, relative energy deficiency in sport (RED-S) [43]. The development of the term RED-S had three main purposes: (1) to draw awareness to the fact that energy restriction can have negative consequences in men in addition to women; (2) to highlight other potential negative health and performance consequences of low energy availability in athletes besides bone problems, and (3) to encourage expansive research into the potential myriad effects of low energy availability in various populations, including Paralympic athletes. Multiple studies have not found evidence of decreased BMD in male athletes with decreased testosterone [1, 16, 21], while other studies have shown decreased BMD in male runners [44] and horse-racing jockeys [45].

Additionally, our group studied hormone levels and DXA-derived BMD in collegiate, male runners, wrestlers, and golfers [46]. Wrestlers had significantly greater BMD at all measured sites than runners and golfers, who were not significantly different from each other. Total and free testosterone levels were not significantly different among the groups, nor were they predictors of BMD at the hip or spine. However, total and free estradiol levels were higher in wrestlers than in runners and were important positive determinants of BMD [46]. Perhaps the failure of prior work to show a correlation among energy availability, testosterone, and low BMD may be secondary to the focus on androgens rather than estrogens. Further work is needed to better understand RED-S and possible effects of estradiol and bone in male athletes.

Fertility

Studies evaluating intense training in men have shown that the inhibition of the HPG axis could manifest as changes in fertility. Some studies have found changes in semen from exercise, noting decreases in sperm motility, quality and number [17, 19, 47, 48], while others have not found such alterations [49, 50]. In the previously mentioned study by Safarinejad et al. [38], those participants assigned to high-intensity training had significantly decreased sperm count, concentration, and motility at 24 weeks of exercise, which worsened through the exercise intervention. Similarly, Vaamonde et al. [51] evaluated untrained subjects after 2 weeks of exhaustive endurance exercise and found negative changes in sperm, FSH, and LH that returned to normal 2–3 days after resuming their baseline exercise habits. Additionally, De Souza et al. [19] showed a negative correlation of volume of exercise with sperm motility and density. The above studies, however, did not control for energy availability. Thus, like much of the work in female athletes, research in male athletes will be more easily interpretable in the future if energy availability is accurately quantified and factored into the analysis.

Females

Acute Changes in Testosterone and Estradiol

In females, short-term consequences of training on the HPG axis have not been as widely studied as in males. Differences in hormonal responses between the sexes are believed to be dependent on basal hormone concentrations (i.e. sex differences in basal estradiol and testosterone) [52]. Cumming et al. [53] studied 7 women (aged 18–21 years) and noted increases in total testosterone after an acute bout of resistance training. In a larger study, Nindl et al. [54] studied hormonal changes after acute bouts of resistance exercise in 47 women (mean age 22 ± 3 years), and also found increases in both free and total testosterone. There have been mixed results pertaining to the effects of a few weeks to a few months of resistance training on basal levels of testosterone in women. Kraemer et al. [55] studied 8 women during 8 weeks of heavy resistance exercise and found a small, but significant elevation in testosterone before exercise by week 6 compared to week 1. Studies have also shown an increase in testosterone with acute bouts of endurance exercise [56, 57].

Studies evaluating acute changes in estradiol are challenging given that estradiol levels change widely during a typical menstrual cycle. Estradiol increases during the follicular phase, peaks prior to ovulation, plummets during ovulation, and then experiences a gradual increase and decrease prior to its nadir in early menses. Estradiol levels also experience a diurnal and ultradian rhythm throughout each day that additionally varies throughout the cycle [58]. Nevertheless, multiple studies have found an acute increase in estradiol immediately after exercise [59, 60]. This increase in estradiol seems to be responsible for greater lipid and less carbohydrate oxidation compared to men during exercise [61, 62]. Estradiol also seems to be protective for muscles during the stress of exercise [63, 64]. While the exact mechanisms are poorly understood, the positive effects of exercise may be exerted by estrogen acting as (1) an antioxidant, therefore minimizing oxidative damage; (2) a membrane stabilizer by inserting itself among phospholipids in the cell membrane, and (3) an estrogen receptor substrate, thus affecting downstream gene regulation and other targets [65].

Female Athlete Triad

The long-term impact of exercise and training on hormone levels has been more widely studied in females, particularly in the setting of decreased energy availability. As mentioned briefly above, the Triad is a combination of decreased energy availability, menstrual irregularity (luteal phase defects, anovulation, oligomenorrhea, and hypothalamic amenorrhea), and poor bone health (decreased BMD and higher risk of fracture) [66, 67]. Lower energy availability from increased caloric expenditure and/or relatively decreased caloric intake leads to a suppression of the HPG axis, diverting energy away from the reproductive system to more vital bodily processes, such as cell maintenance and immune function. GnRH pulsatility is disrupted, leading to changes in more downstream hormonal signaling and functional hypothalamic amenorrhea [66]. Functional hypothalamic amenorrhea is defined as the absence of menses secondary to the suppression of the HPG axis where other causes have been excluded [68]. There is evidence of variable susceptibility to functional hypothalamic amenorrhea based on genetic factors [69]. Estradiol and other hormones affected by low energy availability, including IGF-1, cortisol, and leptin, are important for bone metabolism. Therefore, decreases in energy availability can have negative effects on BMD through multiple pathways [70].

Amenorrhea has been reported in up to 66% of athletes, depending on the sports population studied and how screening was performed [66, 71, 72]. GnRH has a direct effect on the pattern of LH release, and LH pulsatility is a direct reflection of GnRH pulsatility. In one study, alterations in LH release were described in 78% of athletes with amenorrhea [73]. When evaluating secretion of LH in amenorrheic athletes, eumenorrheic athletes, and nonathletic controls aged 14–21 years, overnight secretory LH pulse height, total pulsatile secretion, and area under the concentration time curve (AUC) were lower in athletes with amenorrhea versus nonathletes [74]. In a study examining LH pulsatility in eumenorrheic, sedentary women, subjects were energy restricted from diet alone versus those energy restricted predominantly by increasing exercise. Changes in LH pulse frequency and amplitude were noted in both energy-restricted states, but LH pulse frequency was less decreased when equivalent energy deficiency was achieved mostly from exercise [75]. This suggests that energy restriction, or decreased energy availability, is likely a more important factor in GnRH and LH disruption in Triad, rather than the stress of exercise.

FSH stimulates granulosa cells of the ovaries, which leads to inhibin B secretion and subsequent inhibition of further FSH production, thus allowing only the most advanced (or dominant) follicle to continue to develop and proceed to ovulation. When estradiol levels decrease at the end of the cycle, FSH levels start to rise again and allow for new follicles to be recruited. Although FSH is highly regulated by GnRH, the literature has failed to demonstrate significant differences in FSH levels in athletes with amenorrhea versus eumenorrheic athletes. This may be partially explained by the methods used to study such levels and the significant variability in hormone levels even in eumenorrheic athletes. For example, in a study of daily urinary hormone levels over 3 months in recreational runners who had regular monthly menses, only 45% of the cycles were ovulatory, 43% had luteal phase defects (e.g. shortened luteal phases), and 12% were anovulatory. In this study that involved very careful assessment of gonadotropins and other hormones, FSH elevation during the luteal-follicular transition was lower in athletes with luteal phase defects versus athletes with ovulatory cycles and nonexercising, sedentary controls [76]. Unfortunately, most other studies examining FSH levels in athletes have not gathered samples over multiple times points in one cycle nor have they tested contiguous cycles in subjects.

In a study of 30 women with functional hypothalamic amenorrhea, only 29% had low FSH levels (5th percentile of early follicular phase control values), which was associated with a lower follicular number. However, when 79% of amenorrheic subjects with FSH levels and follicular numbers similar to controls were further studied, some of their functional follicular markers were abnormal. These included higher anti-Müllerian hormone levels, higher anti-Müllerian: 2–5 mm follicular number ratios and lower mean inhibin B levels compared to controls. This suggests that even with 'normal' FSH levels, the terminal growth and function of antral follicles may be affected [77].

It is well established that estradiol levels are lower in amenorrheic athletes with functional hypothalamic amenorrhea or Triad compared to eumenorrheic athletes [78, 79]. Urinary estrone-1-glucuronide (E1G) excretion patterns were studied in women who were categorized by exercise (exercisers or sedentary controls) and menstrual status (ovulatory, luteal phase defects, or anovulatory). While there were no significant differences in peak concentrations of E1G among the groups, the day of peak E1G occurred later in exercisers with luteal phase defects versus exercisers who ovulated. Anovulatory exercisers had lower E1G excretion in the follicular phase compared to sedentary and exercising ovulators, and exercisers with luteal phase defects. E1G AUC was lower in anovulatory exercisers versus sedentary and exercising ovulators during the follicular phase, and exercisers with anovulation or luteal phase defects had lower E1G AUC compared to sedentary ovulators during the luteal phase [80].

Such decreases in estradiol secondary to menstrual irregularity have proven negative effects on BMD, bone microarchitecture, and fracture risk [66, 67, 81]. However, further work has also suggested other negative consequences. Estrogen stimulates the endothelial nitric oxide (NO) synthase signaling system, promoting NO release, which subsequently enhances vascular smooth muscle cell dilation. NO also has anti-atherosclerotic properties [82]. Various researchers have noted endothelial dysfunction in amenorrheic athletes [83–86], with one study noting that estradiol levels correlated positively with vascular function [85] and another noting that the most unfavorable lipid profiles correlated with the most significant menstrual dysfunction in athletes [84]. In the former study, amenorrheic athletes who became eumenorrheic during the follow-up after quitting strenuous athletic activity had improved vascular function that was associated with increased serum estrogen levels [85]. As the IOC's RED-S term suggests, there certainly may be other effects of decreased energy availability on athletes in addition to poor bone health, and more work is needed to explore other potential effects of low estradiol on athletes' health and performance.

Progesterone release is stimulated by LH and has enhanced effects under the influence of estrogens. This is a progestational hormone, because it enhances vascularization of the endometrial cell lining for implantation during the luteal phase of the menstrual cycle and maintains it during pregnancy. Like estradiol, there is evidence that this hormone is also reduced in some female athletes [87]. While the clinical definitions of luteal phase defects have been controversial, they all include low progesterone levels in the luteal phase. Such hormone alterations have negative effects on fertility, secondary to poor follicular development, poor implantation, and pregnancy maintenance (spontaneous abortion) [88].

Energy status is correlated with body fat mass. Adipocytes are responsible for the secretion of leptin and adiponectin, which, as mentioned earlier, have opposing effects on the HPG axis [89–92]. There is consistent evidence that amenorrheic athletes with normal lean body mass and BMI have lower body fat and percent body fat than eumenorrheic athletes and nonathletes [93, 94]. Leptin, an anorexigenic hormone, declines with low energy availability [95, 96] and, as expected, is lower in amenorrheic athletes compared to eumenorrheic athletes and nonathletes [74, 93]. Conversely, there is evidence that adiponectin increases with reduced energy [89, 91]; however, findings in amenorrheic athletes are inconsistent. There were no significant differences in adiponectin levels in adolescent amenorrheic versus eumenorrheic athletes [97], but in another study, adult amenorrheic athletes were found to have higher adiponectin levels than eumenorrheic athletes [98]. Additionally, fat mass plays an important role in the regulation of ghrelin, cortisol, IGF-1, and peptide YY, which in turn affect GnRH regulation [74, 92–94; see also this vol., pp. 1–11, 12–26, 44–57].

Treatment of the Triad should start with modest exercise reduction (10–20%) and an increase in energy availability to at least 30–45 kcal/kg of fat-free mass per day. If the patient is not compliant with treatment, removal from competition may be necessary [41, 66]. Recovery of menstrual cycles and fertility, and improvement in BMD is possible in those athletes who normalize their energy availability. Often BMD cannot improve to a normal range if the energy depletion occurred during adolescence, a time characterized by significant bone accrual, and/or if the decreased energy availability and menstrual dysfunction were prolonged [66, 99, 100]. Pharmacological therapy with oral contraceptive pills (OCPs) with estrogen and progestin has shown inconclusive results despite their widespread use in amenorrheic athletes and patients with anorexia nervosa [41, 101–103]. Unlike OCPs, estrogen delivered via transdermal patches has minimal suppressive effects on the bone trophic hormone, IGF-1, which may contribute to an increase in BMD in amenorrheic athletes not seen with oral estrogen preparations [104]. Our group found an increase in spine and hip BMD with physiological estrogen replacement using a transdermal patch and cyclic oral micronized progesterone in patients with anorexia nervosa [105]. This treatment is currently being tested in amenorrheic athletes. Additionally, further long-term research is needed to determine the lasting effects on fertility and possible treatment of athletes who have suffered prolonged menstrual dysfunction.

Androgens

Androgen levels have been studied to some extent in female athletes. In a large study of 849 elite female athletes competing in the 2011 International Association of Athletics Federations (IAAF) World Championships, blood samples were drawn to determine karyotype and hormone levels [106]. Five subjects were excluded because of doping and 5 subjects were found to be 46XY with disorders in sex development. The prevalence of the genetic 46XY finding in this population (7.1 per 1,000) was 140 times higher than predicted in the general population, thus suggesting a potential selection bias for these individuals to participate in sport [106]. Two previous studies also found a high prevalence of the 46XY karyotype in phenotypic females in the 1992 (7.5 per 1,000) and 1996 Olympic games (2.67 per 1,000) [106, 107]. Notably, in the 2011 IAAF study and in prior reports, genetic testing was only done in those athletes suspected of hyperandrogenism (HA), and, therefore, the prevalence of Y-chromosomal material may be even higher in elite female athletes. However, after excluding known 46XY and doping subjects, a great variability in the hormonal profile was found in different sports at the IAAF Championships. A higher level of testosterone and dehydroepiandrosterone (DHEA) sulfate was seen in throwers and sprinters compared to long-distance runners [106]. When examined according to menstrual status, oligomenorrheic and amenorrheic athletes had lower testosterone and DHEA sulfate, and higher SHBG concentrations than eumenorrheic athletes [106]. These findings were similar to two prior cross-sectional studies; one in adult and one in adolescent female athletes. Both found decreased testosterone levels in amenorrheic compared with eumenorrheic athletes [87, 93].

Rickenlund et al. [108] found that 8 of 25 endurance athletes with oligo- or amenorrhea had significantly higher serum levels of free and total testosterone, androstenedione and LH:FSH ratio, and lower SHBG compared to eumenorrheic endurance athletes and nonathletes. Subsequently, the same authors compared age- and BMI-matched groups of amenorrheic endurance athletes, oligomenorrheic endurance athletes, eumenorrheic athletes, and sedentary controls, and found that oligomenorrheic (but not amenorrheic) athletes had higher levels of diurnal testosterone [109]. They also noted a positive association between 24-hour testosterone and menarchal age [109]. In a recent, small, retrospective cohort study, Javed et al. [110] examined BMI-matched female athletes diagnosed with functional hypothalamic amenorrhea from exercise (FHA-EX) plus clinical or biochemical HA (FHA-EX+HA) versus athletes with FHA-EX only versus females with functional hypothalamic amenorrhea from anorexia nervosa (FHA-AN). Based on the Rotterdam criteria, all subjects in the FHA-EX+HA group met criteria for polycystic ovary syndrome. FHA-EX+HA had significantly higher total testosterone levels compared to FHA-EX, but not compared to FHA-AN. FHA-EX+HA had a higher LH:FSH ratio, higher diastolic blood pressure, and fewer stress fractures compared to the other two groups, and higher fasting glucose and lumbar BMD compared to FHA-EX. In a cross-sectional study of Swedish Olympic athletes, of the few with menstrual disturbances not on hormonal contraception, 1 of 5 amenorrheic athletes and 5 of 8 oligomenorrheic athletes were diagnosed with polycystic ovary syndrome instead of hypothalamic inhibition [111]. There seems to be a positive effect of HA on performance in female athletes and, therefore, a positive selection towards sports [108]. The above studies remind us that there may be overt differences in the genetics of some athletes competing as phenotypic females in addition to subtle metabolic differences in those with mild HA features. In studies determining normal ranges of hormones in healthy, nondoping athletes, in addition to studies of the effects of hypothalamic amenorrhea and Triad on health and performance parameters, it is important to remember the wide range of genetic and metabolic differences that may exist.

Effects of the Menstrual Cycle and Oral Contraceptives on Exercise and Training

Multiple studies have examined the effect of the menstrual cycle on VO_{2max}, aerobic endurance, and anaerobic performance, and most have not found significant differences during the different phases of the cycle [112–115]. One exception was a study of 16 eumenorrheic athletes tested in the early follicular and mid-luteal phases of the menstrual cycle. Both absolute and relative VO_{2max} were slightly lower in the luteal versus follicular phase. However, the cycle phase did not significantly affect maximum heart rate, maximum minute ventilation, maximum respiratory exchange ratio, anaerobic performance, endurance time to fatigue, or isokinetic strength [116]. Similarly, in a study of 8 eumenorrheic athletes studied during the follicular and the luteal phase, subjects finished a cycling distance significantly faster during the follicular phase than the luteal phase. Interestingly, when glucose ingestion was allowed during the distance trial, the time to completion was faster compared to both follicular and luteal phases without carbohydrate ingestion, and there was no difference between the menstrual phases. Thus, proper fueling may negate any small performance differences noted between menstrual phases [117].

Progesterone and synthetic progestins are known to have a central thermogenic effect. An increase in body temperature of 0.3–0.5°C has been noted during pregnancy and the luteal phase of the menstrual cycle. There is associated altered skin blood flow and an increased threshold for cutaneous vasodilation and the onset of sweating. A higher core body temperature may reduce the safe margin for heat accumulation when exercising in a hot, humid environment, potentially decreasing the time to fatigue and compromising performance [118–120].

The effect of exogenous estradiol and progesterone administration on performance has now been widely studied. Studies in the 1980s and 1990s did not find any difference in aerobic performance between OCP users and nonusers [121–124]. More recent studies have found a decrease in VO_{2max} with continued OCP use [125, 126]. In 2013, Joyce et al. [127] evaluated the effects of OCP use on endurance performance and found a decrease in VO_{2max} in OCP users but no changes in endurance performance. Another similar study in rowers did not find a difference between performance among OCP users and nonusers [128]. Notably, some athletes feel better during specific times of their menstrual cycles, suggesting individual variation in performance based on symptoms. To tease out the effects of menstruation and OCPs on performance, much larger studies are needed with reliable hormonal assays, a variety of OCP formulations, and in-depth questioning about training, mood, menstrual symptoms, and more.

Conclusions

The bulk of the literature regarding hormone levels in male athletes focuses on the effects of short bouts of exercise on transient changes in hormone levels. Testosterone has been the hormone most classically examined, because of its positive effects on muscle and strength, and because it is the primary male sex hormone. Overall, effects of long-term training on hormone levels have been less well studied in males and most prior work has not controlled for energy availability, thus confounding results, particularly in endurance athletes. Decreased energy availability in male athletes and its long-term effects need further evaluation. On the other hand, it is well established that decreased energy availability in female athletes suppresses the HPG axis, manifesting as an alteration in the menstrual cycle and decreased BMD. A better understanding is necessary of possible effects of decreased energy availability on performance and other end points. Effects of short-term bouts of exercise on the HPG axis in females include increases in testosterone and estrogen. Such increases are dependent on the timing of the menstrual cycle, energy availability, and the type of exercise. Further studies over the course of multiple menstrual cycles, appropriately controlled for energy availability, are needed to better understand both acute and long-term hormonal responses to exercise and training.

References

1 Hagmar M, Berglund B, Brismar K, Hirschberg AL: Body composition and endocrine profile of male Olympic athletes striving for leanness. Clin J Sport Med 2013;23:197–201.
2 Di Luigi L, Romanelli F, Sgrò P, Lenzi A: Andrological aspects of physical exercise and sport medicine. Endocrine 2012;42:278–284.
3 Melmed S, Williams RH: Williams Textbook of Endocrinology, ed 12. Philadelphia, Elsevier/Saunders, 2011, xviii, p 1897.
4 Vingren JL, Kraemer WJ, Ratamess NA, Anderson JM, Volek JS, Maresh CM: Testosterone physiology in resistance exercise and training: the up-stream regulatory elements. Sports Med 2010;40:1037–1053.
5 Crewther BT, Cook C, Cardinale M, Weatherby RP, Lowe T: Two emerging concepts for elite athletes: the short-term effects of testosterone and cortisol on the neuromuscular system and the dose-response training role of these endogenous hormones. Sports Med 2011;41:103–123.
6 Friedl KE, Dettori JR, Hannan CJ Jr, Patience TH, Plymate SR: Comparison of the effects of high dose testosterone and 19-nortestosterone to a replacement dose of testosterone on strength and body composition in normal men. J Steroid Biochem Mol Biol 1991;40:607–612.
7 Bhasin S, Woodhouse L, Casaburi R, Singh AB, Bhasin D, Berman N, et al: Testosterone dose-response relationships in healthy young men. Am J Physiol Endocrinol Metab 2001;281:E1172–E1181.

8 Sinha-Hikim I, Cornford M, Gaytan H, Lee ML, Bhasin S: Effects of testosterone supplementation on skeletal muscle fiber hypertrophy and satellite cells in community-dwelling older men. J Clin Endocrinol Metab 2006;91:3024–3033.
9 Storer TW, Magliano L, Woodhouse L, Lee ML, Dzekov C, Dzekov J, et al: Testosterone dose-dependently increases maximal voluntary strength and leg power, but does not affect fatigability or specific tension. J Clin Endocrinol Metab 2003;88:1478–1485.
10 Bhasin S, Storer TW, Berman N, Callegari C, Clevenger B, Phillips J, et al: The effects of supraphysiologic doses of testosterone on muscle size and strength in normal men. N Engl J Med 1996;335:1–7.
11 Rogerson S, Weatherby RP, Deakin GB, Meir RA, Coutts RA, Zhou S, et al: The effect of short-term use of testosterone enanthate on muscular strength and power in healthy young men. J Strength Cond Res 2007;21:354–361.
12 Blazevich AJ, Giorgi A: Effect of testosterone administration and weight training on muscle architecture. Med Sci Sports Exerc 2001;33:1688–1693.
13 Fahrner CL, Hackney AC: Effects of endurance exercise on free testosterone concentration and the binding affinity of sex hormone binding globulin (SHBG). Int J Sports Med 1998;19:12–15.
14 Grandys M, Majerczak J, Duda K, Zapart-Bukowska J, Kulpa J, Zoladz JA: Endurance training of moderate intensity increases testosterone concentration in young, healthy men. Int J Sports Med 2009;30:489–495.
15 Fitzgerald LZ, Robbins WA, Kesner JS, Xun L: Reproductive hormones and interleukin-6 in serious leisure male athletes. Eur J Appl Physiol 2012;112:3765–3773.
16 MacKelvie KJ, Taunton JE, McKay HA, Khan KM: Bone mineral density and serum testosterone in chronically trained, high mileage 40-55 year old male runners. Br J Sports Med 2000;34:273–278.
17 Lucia A, Chicharro JL, Pérez M, Serratosa L, Bandrés F, Legido JC: Reproductive function in male endurance athletes: sperm analysis and hormonal profile. J Appl Physiol (1985) 1996;81:2627–2636.
18 Saka T, Sofikerim M, Demirtas A, Kulaksizoglu S, Caniklioglu M, Karacagil M: Rigorous bicycling does not increase serum levels of total and free prostate-specific antigen (PSA), the free/total PSA ratio, gonadotropin levels, or uroflowmetric parameters. Urology 2009;74:1325–1330.
19 De Souza MJ, Arce JC, Pescatello LS, Scherzer HS, Luciano AA: Gonadal hormones and semen quality in male runners. A volume threshold effect of endurance training. Int J Sports Med 1994;15:383–391.
20 Wheeler GD, Wall SR, Belcastro AN, Cumming DC: Reduced serum testosterone and prolactin levels in male distance runners. JAMA 1984;252:514–516.
21 Maïmoun L, Lumbroso S, Manetta J, Paris F, Leroux JL, Sultan C: Testosterone is significantly reduced in endurance athletes without impact on bone mineral density. Horm Res 2003;59:285–292.
22 Hackney AC, Fahrner CL, Gulledge TP: Basal reproductive hormonal profiles are altered in endurance trained men. J Sports Med Phys Fitness 1998;38:138–141.
23 Arce JC, De Souza MJ, Pescatello LS, Luciano AA: Subclinical alterations in hormone and semen profile in athletes. Fertil Steril 1993;59:398–404.
24 Grasso G, Lodi L, Lupo C, Muscettola M: Glucocorticoid receptors in human peripheral blood mononuclear cells in relation to age and to sport activity. Life Sci 1997;61:301–308.
25 Izquierdo M, Ibáñez J, Häkkinen K, Kraemer WJ, Ruesta M, Gorostiaga EM: Maximal strength and power, muscle mass, endurance and serum hormones in weightlifters and road cyclists. J Sports Sci 2004;22:465–478.
26 Maestu J, Eliakim A, Jürimäe J, Valter I, Jürimäe T: Anabolic and catabolic hormones and energy balance of the male bodybuilders during the preparation for the competition. J Strength Cond Res 2010;24:1074–1081.
27 Grandys M, Majerczak J, Zapart-Bukowska J, Kulpa J, Zoladz JA: Gonadal hormone status in highly trained sprinters and in untrained men. J Strength Cond Res 2011;25:1079–1084.
28 Pullinen T, Mero A, MacDonald E, Pakarinen A, Komi PV: Plasma catecholamine and serum testosterone responses to four units of resistance exercise in young and adult male athletes. Eur J Appl Physiol Occup Physiol 1998;77:413–420.
29 Pullinen T, Mero A, Huttunen P, Pakarinen A, Komi PV: Resistance exercise-induced hormonal responses in men, women, and pubescent boys. Med Sci Sports Exerc 2002;34:806–813.
30 Fahey TD, Rolph R, Moungmee P, Nagel J, Mortara S: Serum testosterone, body composition, and strength of young adults. Med Sci Sports 1976;8:31–34.
31 Kraemer WJ, Fry AC, Warren BJ, Stone MH, Fleck SJ, Kearney JT, et al: Acute hormonal responses in elite junior weightlifters. Int J Sports Med 1992;13:103–109.
32 Gurd B, Klentrou P: Physical and pubertal development in young male gymnasts. J Appl Physiol (1985) 2003;95:1011–1015.
33 Moore SA, Moore M, Klentrou P, Sullivan P, Falk B: Maturity status in male child and adolescent athletes. J Sports Med Phys Fitness 2010;50:486–493.

34 Häkkinen K, Pakarinen A, Kraemer WJ, Newton RU, Alen M: Basal concentrations and acute responses of serum hormones and strength development during heavy resistance training in middle-aged and elderly men and women. J Gerontol A Biol Sci Med Sci 2000;55:B95–B105.
35 Di Luigi L, Sgrò P, Fierro V, Bianchini S, Battistini G, Magini V, Jannini EA, Lenzi A: Prevalence of undiagnosed testosterone deficiency in aging athletes: does exercise training influence the symptoms of male hypogonadism? J Sex Med 2010;7:2591–2601.
36 Healy ML, Gibney J, Pentecost C, Wheeler MJ, Sonksen PH: Endocrine profiles in 693 elite athletes in the postcompetition setting. Clin Endocrinol (Oxf) 2014;81:294–305.
37 Meeusen R, Duclos M, Foster C, Fry A, Gleeson M, Nieman D, et al: Prevention, diagnosis, and treatment of the overtraining syndrome: joint consensus statement of the European College of Sport Science and the American College of Sports Medicine. Med Sci Sports Exerc 2013;45:186–205.
38 Safarinejad MR, Azma K, Kolahi AA: The effects of intensive, long-term treadmill running on reproductive hormones, hypothalamus-pituitary-testis axis, and semen quality: a randomized controlled study. J Endocrinol 2009;200:259–271.
39 Hagmar M, Hirschberg AL, Berglund L, Berglund B: Special attention to the weight-control strategies employed by Olympic athletes striving for leanness is required. Clin J Sport Med 2008;18:5–9.
40 Martinsen M, Bratland-Sanda S, Eriksson AK, Sundgot-Borgen J: Dieting to win or to be thin? A study of dieting and disordered eating among adolescent elite athletes and non-athlete controls. Br J Sports Med 2010;44:70–76.
41 De Souza MJ, Nattiv A, Joy E, Misra M, Williams NI, Mallinson RJ, et al: 2014 Female Athlete Triad Coalition Consensus Statement on Treatment and Return to Play of the Female Athlete Triad: 1st International Conference held in San Francisco, California, May 2012, and 2nd International Conference held in Indianapolis, Indiana, May 2013. Br J Sports Med 2014;48:289.
42 Misra M, Katzman DK, Cord J, Manning SJ, Mendes N, Herzog DB, et al: Bone metabolism in adolescent boys with anorexia nervosa. J Clin Endocrinol Metab 2008;93:3029–3036.
43 Mountjoy M, Sundgot-Borgen J, Burke L, Carter S, Constantini N, Lebrun C, et al: The IOC consensus statement: beyond the female athlete triad – relative energy deficiency in sport (RED-S). Br J Sports Med 2014;48:491–497.
44 Hind K, Truscott JG, Evans JA: Low lumbar spine bone mineral density in both male and female endurance runners. Bone 2006;39:880–885.
45 Dolan E, McGoldrick A, Davenport C, Kelleher G, Byrne B, Tormey W, et al: An altered hormonal profile and elevated rate of bone loss are associated with low bone mass in professional horse-racing jockeys. J Bone Miner Metab 2012;30:534–542.
46 Ackerman KE, Skrinar GS, Medvedova E, Misra M, Miller KK: Estradiol levels predict bone mineral density in male collegiate athletes: a pilot study. Clin Endocrinol (Oxf) 2012;76:339–345.
47 Roberts AC, McClure RD, Weiner RI, Brooks GA: Overtraining affects male reproductive status. Fertil Steril 1993;60:686–692.
48 Gebreegziabher Y, Marcos E, McKinon W, Rogers G: Sperm characteristics of endurance trained cyclists. Int J Sports Med 2004;25:247–251.
49 Ayers JW, Komesu Y, Romani T, Ansbacher R: Anthropomorphic, hormonal, and psychologic correlates of semen quality in endurance-trained male athletes. Fertil Steril 1985;43:917–921.
50 Bagatell CJ, Bremner WJ: Sperm counts and reproductive hormones in male marathoners and lean controls. Fertil Steril 1990;53:688–692.
51 Vaamonde D, Da Silva ME, Poblador MS, Lancho JL: Reproductive profile of physically active men after exhaustive endurance exercise. Int J Sports Med 2006;27:680–689.
52 Häkkinen K, Häkkinen A: Neuromuscular adaptations during intensive strength training in middle-aged and elderly males and females. Electromyogr Clin Neurophysiol 1995;35:137–147.
53 Cumming DC, Wall SR, Galbraith MA, Belcastro AN: Reproductive hormone responses to resistance exercise. Med Sci Sports Exerc 1987;19:234–238.
54 Nindl BC, Kraemer WJ, Gotshalk LA, Marx JO, Volek JS, Bush FA, et al: Testosterone responses after resistance exercise in women: influence of regional fat distribution. Int J Sport Nutr Exerc Metab 2001;11:451–465.
55 Kraemer WJ, Staron RS, Hagerman FC, Hikida RS, Fry AC, Gordon SE, et al: The effects of short-term resistance training on endocrine function in men and women. Eur J Appl Physiol Occup Physiol 1998;78:69–76.
56 Consitt LA, Copeland JL, Tremblay MS: Hormone responses to resistance vs. endurance exercise in premenopausal females. Can J Appl Physiol 2001;26:574–587.
57 Enea C, Boisseau N, Ottavy M, Mulliez J, Millet C, Ingrand I, et al: Effects of menstrual cycle, oral contraception, and training on exercise-induced changes in circulating DHEA-sulphate and testosterone in young women. Eur J Appl Physiol 2009;106:365–373.
58 Bao AM, Liu RY, van Someren EJ, Hofman MA, Cao YX, Zhou JN: Diurnal rhythm of free estradiol during the menstrual cycle. Eur J Endocrinol 2003;148:227–232.

59 Kraemer RR, Heleniak RJ, Tryniecki JL, Kraemer GR, Okazaki NJ, Castracane VD: Follicular and luteal phase hormonal responses to low-volume resistive exercise. Med Sci Sports Exerc 1995;27:809–817.
60 Walberg-Rankin J, Franke WD, Gwazdauskas FC: Response of beta-endorphin and estradiol to resistance exercise in females during energy balance and energy restriction. Int J Sports Med 1992;13:542–547.
61 Carter S, McKenzie S, Mourtzakis M, Mahoney DJ, Tarnopolsky MA: Short-term 17beta-estradiol decreases glucose R(a) but not whole body metabolism during endurance exercise. J Appl Physiol (1985) 2001;90:139–146.
62 Tarnopolsky MA: Sex differences in exercise metabolism and the role of 17-beta estradiol. Med Sci Sports Exerc 2008;40:648–654.
63 Bar PR, Amelink GJ, Oldenburg B, Blankenstein MA: Prevention of exercise-induced muscle membrane damage by oestradiol. Life Sci 1988;42:2677–2681.
64 Komulainen J, Koskinen SO, Kalliokoski R, Takala TE, Vihko V: Gender differences in skeletal muscle fibre damage after eccentrically biased downhill running in rats. Acta Physiol Scand 1999;165:57–63.
65 Enns DL, Tiidus PM: The influence of estrogen on skeletal muscle: sex matters. Sports Med 2010;40:41–58.
66 Nattiv A, Loucks AB, Manore MM, Sanborn CF, Sundgot-Borgen J, Warren MP, et al: American College of Sports Medicine position stand. The female athlete triad. Med Sci Sports Exerc 2007;39:1867–1882.
67 Ackerman KE, Cano Sokoloff N, De Nardo Maffazioli G, Clarke HM, Lee H, Misra M: Fractures in relation to menstrual status and bone parameters in young athletes. Med Sci Sports Exerc 2015;47:1577–1586.
68 Gordon CM: Clinical practice. Functional hypothalamic amenorrhea. N Engl J Med 2010;363:365–371.
69 Caronia LM, Martin C, Welt CK, Sykiotis GP, Quinton R, Thambundit A, et al: A genetic basis for functional hypothalamic amenorrhea. N Engl J Med 2011;364:215–225.
70 Ackerman KE, Misra M: Neuroendocrine abnormalities in female athletes; in Gordon CM, LeBoff M (eds): The Female Athlete Triad. A Clinical Guide. Berlin, Springer, 2014.
71 Nichols JF, Rauh MJ, Lawson MJ, Ji M, Barkai HS: Prevalence of the female athlete triad syndrome among high school athletes. Arch Pediatr Adolesc Med 2006;160:137–142.
72 Hobart JA, Smucker DR: The female athlete triad (review). Am Fam Physician 2000;61:3357–3364, 3367.
73 Perkins RB, Hall JE, Martin KA: Neuroendocrine abnormalities in hypothalamic amenorrhea: spectrum, stability, and response to neurotransmitter modulation. J Clin Endocrinol Metab 1999;84:1905–1911.
74 Ackerman KE, Slusarz K, Guereca G, Pierce L, Slattery M, Mendes N, et al: Higher ghrelin and lower leptin secretion are associated with lower LH secretion in young amenorrheic athletes compared with eumenorrheic athletes and controls. Am J Physiol Endocrinol Metab 2012;302:E800–E806.
75 Loucks AB, Verdun M, Heath EM: Low energy availability, not stress of exercise, alters LH pulsatility in exercising women. J Appl Physiol (1985) 1998;84:37–46.
76 De Souza MJ, Miller BE, Loucks AB, Luciano AA, Pescatello LS, et al: High frequency of luteal phase deficiency and anovulation in recreational women runners: blunted elevation in follicle-stimulating hormone observed during luteal-follicular transition. J Clin Endocrinol Metab 1998;83:4220–4232.
77 Jonard S, Pigny P, Jacquesson L, Demerle-Roux C, Robert Y, Dewailly D: The ovarian markers of the FSH insufficiency in functional hypothalamic amenorrhoea. Hum Reprod 2005;20:101–107.
78 Drinkwater BL, Nilson K, Chesnut CH 3rd, Bremner WJ, Shainholtz S, Southworth MB: Bone mineral content of amenorrheic and eumenorrheic athletes. N Engl J Med 1984;311:277–281.
79 Laughlin GA, Dominguez CE, Yen SS: Nutritional and endocrine-metabolic aberrations in women with functional hypothalamic amenorrhea. J Clin Endocrinol Metab 1998;83:25–32.
80 De Souza MJ, Toombs RJ, Scheid JL, O'Donnell E, West SL, Williams NI: High prevalence of subtle and severe menstrual disturbances in exercising women: confirmation using daily hormone measures. Hum Reprod 2010;25:491–503.
81 Ackerman KE, Nazem T, Chapko D, Russell M, Mendes N, Taylor AP, et al: Bone microarchitecture is impaired in adolescent amenorrheic athletes compared with eumenorrheic athletes and nonathletic controls. J Clin Endocrinol Metab 2011;96:3123–3133.
82 Mendelsohn ME: Estrogen actions in the cardiovascular system. Climacteric 2009;12(suppl 1):18–21.
83 Zeni Hoch A, Dempsey RL, Carrera GF, Wilson CR, Chen EH, Barnabei VM, et al: Is there an association between athletic amenorrhea and endothelial cell dysfunction? Med Sci Sports Exerc 2003;35:377–383.
84 Rickenlund A, Eriksson MJ, Schenck-Gustafsson K, Hirschberg AL: Amenorrhea in female athletes is associated with endothelial dysfunction and unfavorable lipid profile. J Clin Endocrinol Metab 2005;90:1354–1359.

85 Yoshida N, Ikeda H, Sugi K, Imaizumi T: Impaired endothelium-dependent and -independent vasodilation in young female athletes with exercise-associated amenorrhea. Arterioscler Thromb Vasc Biol 2006;26:231–232.
86 Hoch AZ, Papanek P, Szabo A, Widlansky ME, Schimke JE, Gutterman DD: Association between the female athlete triad and endothelial dysfunction in dancers. Clin J Sport Med 2011;21:119–125.
87 Loucks AB, Mortola JF, Girton L, Yen SS: Alterations in the hypothalamic-pituitary-ovarian and the hypothalamic-pituitary-adrenal axes in athletic women. J Clin Endocrinol Metab 1989;68:402–411.
88 De Souza MJ: Menstrual disturbances in athletes: a focus on luteal phase defects. Med Sci Sports Exerc 2003;35:1553–1563.
89 Lu M, Tang Q, Olefsky JM, Mellon PL, Webster NJ: Adiponectin activates adenosine monophosphate-activated protein kinase and decreases luteinizing hormone secretion in LbetaT2 gonadotropes. Mol Endocrinol 2008;22:760–771.
90 Welt CK, Chan JL, Bullen J, Murphy R, Smith P, DePaoli AM, et al: Recombinant human leptin in women with hypothalamic amenorrhea. N Engl J Med 2004;351:987–997.
91 Wen JP, Lv WS, Yang J, Nie AF, Cheng XB, Yang Y, et al: Globular adiponectin inhibits GnRH secretion from GT1-7 hypothalamic GnRH neurons by induction of hyperpolarization of membrane potential. Biochem Biophys Res Commun 2008;371:756–761.
92 Misra M, Miller KK, Cord J, Prabhakaran R, Herzog DB, Goldstein M, et al: Relationships between serum adipokines, insulin levels, and bone density in girls with anorexia nervosa. J Clin Endocrinol Metab 2007;92:2046–2052.
93 Christo K, Cord J, Mendes N, Miller KK, Goldstein MA, Klibanski A, et al: Acylated ghrelin and leptin in adolescent athletes with amenorrhea, eumenorrheic athletes and controls: a cross-sectional study. Clin Endocrinol (Oxf) 2008;69:628–633.
94 Ackerman KE, Patel KT, Guereca G, Pierce L, Herzog DB, Misra M: Cortisol secretory parameters in young exercisers in relation to LH secretion and bone parameters. Clin Endocrinol (Oxf) 2013;78:114–119.
95 Grinspoon S, Gulick T, Askari H, Landt M, Lee K, Anderson E, et al: Serum leptin levels in women with anorexia nervosa. J Clin Endocrinol Metab 1996;81:3861–3863.
96 Grinspoon SK, Askari H, Landt ML, Nathan DM, Schoenfeld DA, Hayden DL, et al: Effects of fasting and glucose infusion on basal and overnight leptin concentrations in normal-weight women. Am J Clin Nutr 1997;66:1352–1356.
97 Russell M, Stark J, Nayak S, Miller KK, Herzog DB, Klibanski A, et al: Peptide YY in adolescent athletes with amenorrhea, eumenorrheic athletes and non-athletic controls. Bone 2009;45:104–109.
98 O'Donnell E, De Souza MJ: Increased serum adiponectin concentrations in amenorrheic physically active women are associated with impaired bone health but not with estrogen exposure. Bone 2011;48:760–767.
99 Keen AD, Drinkwater BL: Irreversible bone loss in former amenorrheic athletes. Osteoporos Int 1997;7:311–315.
100 Arends JC, Cheung MY, Barrack MT, Nattiv A: Restoration of menses with nonpharmacologic therapy in college athletes with menstrual disturbances: a 5-year retrospective study. Int J Sport Nutr Exerc Metab 2012;22:98–108.
101 Miller BE, De Souza MJ, Slade K, Luciano AA: Sublingual administration of micronized estradiol and progesterone, with and without micronized testosterone: effect on biochemical markers of bone metabolism and bone mineral density. Menopause 2000;7:318–326.
102 Vescovi JD, Jamal SA, De Souza MJ: Strategies to reverse bone loss in women with functional hypothalamic amenorrhea: a systematic review of the literature. Osteoporos Int 2008;19:465–478.
103 Bachrach LK: Acquisition of optimal bone mass in childhood and adolescence. Trends Endocrinol Metab 2001;12:22–28.
104 Nazem TG, Ackerman KE: The female athlete triad. Sports Health 2012;4:302–311.
105 Misra M, Katzman D, Miller KK, Mendes N, Snelgrove D, Russell M, et al: Physiologic estrogen replacement increases bone density in adolescent girls with anorexia nervosa. J Bone Miner Res 2011;26:2430–2438.
106 Bermon S, Garnier PY, Hirschberg AL, Robinson N, Giraud S, Nicoli R, et al: Serum androgen levels in elite female athletes. J Clin Endocrinol Metab 2014;99:4328–4335.
107 Fenichel P, Paris F, Philibert P, Hiéronimus S, Gaspari L, Kurzenne JY, et al: Molecular diagnosis of 5α-reductase deficiency in 4 elite young female athletes through hormonal screening for hyperandrogenism. J Clin Endocrinol Metab 2013;98:E1055–E1059.
108 Rickenlund A, Carlström K, Ekblom B, Brismar TB, von Schoultz B, Hirschberg AL: Hyperandrogenicity is an alternative mechanism underlying oligomenorrhea or amenorrhea in female athletes and may improve physical performance. Fertil Steril 2003;79:947–955.

109 Rickenlund A, Thorén M, Carlström K, von Schoultz B, Hirschberg AL: Diurnal profiles of testosterone and pituitary hormones suggest different mechanisms for menstrual disturbances in endurance athletes. J Clin Endocrinol Metab 2004;89:702–707.
110 Javed A, Kashyap R, Lteif AN: Hyperandrogenism in female athletes with functional hypothalamic amenorrhea: a distinct phenotype. Int J Womens Health 2015;7:103–111.
111 Hagmar M, Berglund B, Brismar K, Hirschberg AL: Hyperandrogenism may explain reproductive dysfunction in Olympic athletes. Med Sci Sports Exerc 2009;41:1241–1248.
112 De Souza MJ, Maguire MS, Rubin KR, Maresh CM: Effects of menstrual phase and amenorrhea on exercise performance in runners. Med Sci Sports Exerc 1990;22:575–580.
113 Bemben DA, Salm PC, Salm AJ: Ventilatory and blood lactate responses to maximal treadmill exercise during the menstrual cycle. J Sports Med Phys Fitness 1995;35:257–262.
114 Bushman B, Masterson G, Nelsen J: Anaerobic power performance and the menstrual cycle: eumenorrheic and oral contraceptive users. J Sports Med Phys Fitness 2006;46:132–137.
115 Giacomoni M, Bernard T, Gavarry O, Altare S, Falgairette G: Influence of the menstrual cycle phase and menstrual symptoms on maximal anaerobic performance. Med Sci Sports Exerc 2000;32:486–492.
116 Lebrun CM, McKenzie DC, Prior JC, Taunton JE: Effects of menstrual cycle phase on athletic performance. Med Sci Sports Exerc 1995;27:437–444.
117 Campbell SE, Angus DJ, Febbraio MA: Glucose kinetics and exercise performance during phases of the menstrual cycle: effect of glucose ingestion. Am J Physiol Endocrinol Metab 2001;281:E817–E825.
118 Constantini NW, Dubnov G, Lebrun CM: The menstrual cycle and sport performance. Clin Sports Med 2005;24:e51–e82, xiii–xiv.
119 Charkoudian N, Johnson JM: Female reproductive hormones and thermoregulatory control of skin blood flow. Exerc Sport Sci Rev 2000;28:108–112.
120 Janse DE Jonge XA, Thompson MW, Chuter VH, Silk LN, Thom JM: Exercise performance over the menstrual cycle in temperate and hot, humid conditions. Med Sci Sports Exerc 2012;44:2190–2198.
121 McNeill AW, Mozingo E: Changes in the metabolic cost of standardized work associated with the use of an oral contraceptive. J Sports Med Phys Fitness 1981;21:238–244.
122 Huisveld IA, Hospers JE, Bernink MJ, Erich WB, Bouma BN: The effect of oral contraceptives and exercise on hemostatic and fibrinolytic mechanisms in trained women. Int J Sports Med 1983;4:97–103.
123 Bryner RW, Toffle RC, Ullrich IH, Yeater RA: Effect of low dose oral contraceptives on exercise performance. Br J Sports Med 1996;30:36–40.
124 Lynch NJ, Nimmo MA: Effects of menstrual cycle phase and oral contraceptive use on intermittent exercise. Eur J Appl Physiol Occup Physiol 1998;78:565–572.
125 Casazza GA, Suh SH, Miller BF, Navazio FM, Brooks GA: Effects of oral contraceptives on peak exercise capacity. J Appl Physiol (1985) 2002;93:1698–1702.
126 Lebrun CM, Petit MA, McKenzie DC, Taunton JE, Prior JC: Decreased maximal aerobic capacity with use of a triphasic oral contraceptive in highly active women: a randomised controlled trial. Br J Sports Med 2003;37:315–320.
127 Joyce S, Sabapathy S, Bulmer A, Minahan C: Effect of long-term oral contraceptive use on determinants of endurance performance. J Strength Cond Res 2013;27:1891–1896.
128 Vaiksaar S, Jürimäe J, Mäestu J, Purge P, Kalytka S, Shakhlina L, et al: No effect of menstrual cycle phase and oral contraceptive use on endurance performance in rowers. J Strength Cond Res 2011;25:1571–1578.

Natalia Cano Sokoloff, MD
55 Fruit Street
BUL 457B
Boston, MA 02114 (USA)
E-Mail natalia.cano@gmail.com

Lanfranco F, Strasburger CJ (eds): Sports Endocrinology.
Front Horm Res. Basel, Karger, 2016, vol 47, pp 44–57 (DOI: 10.1159/000445156)

Metabolic Effects of Exercise

Paolo Moghetti · Elisabetta Bacchi · Corinna Brangani · Silvia Donà · Carlo Negri

Division of Endocrinology, Diabetes and Metabolism, Department of Medicine, University of Verona, and Azienda Ospedaliera Universitaria Integrata Verona, Verona, Italy

Abstract

Exercise has a powerful action on metabolism, and adaptation of the body to changes induced by exercise is fundamental to be able to provide the energy required for muscle contraction and physiological functions of vital tissues. Depending on the intensity and duration of exercise, different mechanisms are called on to make energy available, and under homeostatic control, this is guaranteed by rapid and coordinated changes in the secretion of several hormones. Molecular mechanisms controlling muscle function and fiber phenotype are related to the specific mode of muscle activation. We can distinguish between two fundamental types of physical activity, endurance exercise and strength exercise, although there is a continuum between these exercise modalities. Besides the acute changes induced by a single exercise session, regular exercise may induce chronic adaptations, improving exercise capacity and affecting energy metabolism. Notably, although acute metabolic effects of exercise are mostly due to insulin-independent effects, exercise training may improve muscle insulin sensitivity and is considered a key tool in the prevention and treatment of metabolic disorders. This chapter focuses on the biochemistry of energy supply to the exercising muscle, on molecular mechanisms involved and on the physiology of energy metabolism during exercise in healthy subjects and patients with insulin resistance and/or diabetes.

The Biochemistry of Energy Supply to the Exercising Muscle

Exercise is one of the most powerful modulators of metabolism [1]. A 70-kg marathon runner may cover 42 km in less than 130 min. In the meantime, he expends approximately 3,000 kcal, oxidizes 600–700 g of carbohydrates and 30–40 g of fat, utilizes about 600 liters of oxygen, and breaks down and reforms more than 150 mol of adenosine triphosphate (ATP), which weigh about 63 kg [2].

Depending on the intensity and duration of the exercise, different energetic mechanisms are called on to provide energy to muscles and to the whole body. Each energy-requiring process in the cell is made possible by the availability of a unique carrier of free energy: ATP. This molecule is generated by the oxidation of macronutrients (carbohydrates, lipids, and proteins) and used as a common energetic currency, spent to synthesize proteins, transport molecules inside and outside the cells, provide muscle contraction, and ensure tissue growth and maintenance. Even though ATP represents the immediate source to realize energy-dependent processes, its concentration in tissues is quite low: 2–6 mmol/kg. For this reason, cells are able to keep ATP concentrations constant during slow processes such as food oxidation, but not in muscles during the transition from rest to maximal exercise. During a sprint, for example, ATP requirement in the muscle can increase more than 100 times compared to values needed at rest. If not properly and immediately restored, the ATP content of all muscle cells can supply energy for only 2–3 s during high-intensity activity. However, sustained exercise is made possible by the fact that hydrolyzed ATP is immediately resynthesized. The rate of ATP hydrolysis during maximal exercise may be as high as 0.5 kg/min [3].

ATP can be resynthesized from ADP through three different ways: (a) by phosphocreatine (PCr; alactic anaerobic system); (b) by anaerobic glycolysis (lactic anaerobic system), and (c) by oxidative phosphorylation (aerobic system).

Phosphocreatine System

To avoid immediate ATP consumption during maximal muscle contraction, another intracellular high-energy phosphate compound, PCr, is able to quickly restore ATP.

In humans, 92–96% of total PCr of the body is stored in skeletal muscles, and its concentration is 3–4 times higher than that of ATP (18–20 mmol/kg muscle). PCr transfers its phosphate to ADP to create ATP and creatine, and this process is catalyzed by creatine kinase [2]:

$$\text{ADP} + \text{PCr} + \text{H}^+ \leftrightarrow \text{ATP} + \text{Cr}.$$

This pathway is also called alactic anaerobic, because it does not require oxygen and does not lead to lactate production. PCr is the major ATP donor during the first seconds of intense physical activity.

Glycolytic Pathway

If maximal effort continues, beyond 10 s, energy for continual ATP resynthesis must originate from less-rapid catabolism of the stored macronutrients: triacylglycerol and glycogen molecules stored within muscle cells, blood glucose (derived from liver glycogen during fasting), free fatty acids (FFA; derived from triacylglycerol stored in liver and adipocytes), and intramuscular and liver-derived carbon skeletons of amino acids [4].

Carbohydrates are the only macronutrients able to provide ATP anaerobically, especially during maximal exercise. The first step of glucose degradation is a series of fermentation reactions called glycolysis. In muscle metabolism, there are two starting substances for the glycolytic pathway: glucose and glycogen. Glycogen is easily available in muscles and can be quickly used to fuel glycolysis. Both glucose (a) and glycogen (b) generate the same products; the only difference is that a glucose unit from glycogen produces one more net ATP than a free glucose unit [2]:

(a) Glucose + 2 ADP + 2 Pi + 2 NAD^+
→ 2 pyruvate + 2 ATP + 2 NADH + 2 H^+
(b) $Glycogen_n$ + 3 ADP + 3 Pi + 2 NAD^+
→ $glycogen_{n-1}$ + 2 pyruvate + 3 ATP + 2 NADH + H^+.

Pyruvate obtained by glycolysis has two main metabolic fates: it can be oxidized within the mitochondrion in the oxidative phosphorylation process or converted into lactate by the enzyme lactate dehydrogenase:

Pyruvate + NADH + H^+ ↔ lactate + NAD^+.

When pyruvate is converted into lactate, the whole process (from glycogen or glucose to lactate) is called anaerobic glycolysis, because of the absence of oxygen in ATP production. Conversely, when pyruvate enters a mitochondrion, it is metabolized to carbon dioxide and water; the entire process is called aerobic glycolysis because it requires oxygen. Pyruvate oxidation is a rich source of ATP: every glucose unit can produce two pyruvate molecules and their complete oxidation supplies 25 ATP molecules [2].

The regeneration of NAD^+ (in the reduction of pyruvate to lactate) sustains continued glycolysis under anaerobic conditions. If NAD^+ were not regenerated, glycolysis could not proceed [5].

Anaerobic glycolysis is a characteristic metabolic pathway of fast-twitch muscle fibers, where it can preserve full ATP availability for about the 1st min of activity. The anaerobic reactions of glycolysis release only about 5% of the energy stored within the glucose molecule [4]. In the presence of oxygen, which is mandatory for more protracted muscle contraction, glycolytic reactions occur at a slower rate and participate with a minor contribution to ATP supply [5].

Aerobic Pathway

Much more energy can be extracted aerobically by means of the citric acid cycle (or Krebs cycle) and the electron transport chain (or respiratory chain). The entry point to this oxidative pathway is acetyl coenzyme A (CoA), which may be formed inside mitochondria by the oxidative decarboxylation of pyruvate [5]:

Pyruvate + NAD^+ + CoA → acetyl CoA + CO_2 + NADH.

The acetyl group can be derived from any kind of fuel molecule. Initially, intracellular glycogen and FFA are the main substrates to enter the oxidative pathway. However, if exercise is prolonged, oxidation of circulating glucose and FFA become the prominent ATP source. The contribution of branched-chain amino acids and proteins, in general, to ATP formation during exercise is very limited: <2%; only if glycogen stores are severely depleted can this fraction rise up to 10% [5].

The citric acid cycle produces electrons in the form of reduced coenzymes (mostly NADH). These electrons feed into the electron transport chain and are passed through a series of carriers to oxygen. The addition of electrons to oxygen allows it to combine with two protons (H^+) to produce water. Free energy produced in the electron transport chain is used to phosphorylate ADP to ATP. Acetyl can arise from the breakdown of fatty acids (FAs) using β-oxidation. Acetyl is also produced in mitochondria from pyruvate produced during glycolysis.

The number of ATP moles that can be formed for each mole of fuel oxidized in the cell is thus:

$$C_6H_{12}O_6 + 6\ O_2 + 32(ADP + Pi)$$
$$\rightarrow 6\ CO_2 + 32\ ATP + 38\ H_2O \text{ (glucose);}$$
$$C_{16}H_{32}O_2 + 23\ O_2 + 106(ADP + Pi)$$
$$\rightarrow 16\ CO_2 + 106\ ATP + 122\ H_20 \text{ (palmitic acid, a typical FA).}$$

Molecular Mechanisms Underlying the Metabolic Effects of Exercise

Molecular mechanisms controlling muscle function and fiber phenotype are related to the specific mode of muscle activation. In this regard, we can distinguish between endurance training and strength training, although these two modalities represent the extremes of a continuum of exercise protocols.

Regular endurance exercise results in an increased expression of slower myosin, associated with a fiber-type shift towards the type 1 phenotype. The lag time for these changes may be about 1 week [6]. The fiber cross-sectional area is scarcely affected, whereas muscle capillarity is enhanced, and the number and size of mitochondria increase [7].

Conversely, strength training has a greater effect on the muscle fiber cross-sectional area, mainly due to an increase in the number of myofibrils [8]. Mitochondria and capillarity are little affected.

As the different changes indicate, specific adaptive mechanisms underlie these phenomena.

Endurance Training

There is evidence of transcriptional regulation of several metabolic genes in response to endurance exercise. In this regard, the mRNA of mitochondrial proteins encoded, both at the mitochondrial and at the nuclear level, was found to be increased to a similar extent (1.5- to 1.9-fold).

A number of mechanisms may be involved in initiating this genomic response and may participate in the adaptation to endurance training. The most important ones are listed below:

- ATP consumption, with the subsequent increase in adenosine monophosphate (AMP) production, activates 5′-AMP-activated protein kinase (AMPK) [9]. This multisubstrate serine/threonine kinase directly phosphorylates peroxisome proliferator-activated receptor (PPAR)-γ coactivator 1α (PGC-1α), which is a key activator of the mitochondrial biogenesis program [10].
- Increased cytosolic Ca^{2+} regulates downstream gene expression, mainly through activation of AMPK. An indirect pathway also participates in this process, mediated by calmodulin.
- ROS production, which increases during contractile activity, may contribute to AMPK activation.
- HIF-1 (hypoxia-inducibile factor-1) translocates to the nucleus during cell hypoxic stress, determining PGC-1α, GLUT4, and phosphofructokinase gene activation.
- SIRT1 (silent mating-type information regulator 2 homolog 1) is activated by the increase in substrate (NAD^+) availability and contributes to PGC-1α activation.
- Intramyofibrillar availability of FFAs directly stimulates PPARs, which are molecular sensors of these substrates.

In this series of events, PGC-1α acts as the key downstream element of most signaling pathways responsive to endurance exercise stress. It is considered the master regulator of mitochondrial biogenesis in skeletal muscles, activating the synthesis of all proteins necessary for replication and transcription of mitochondrial DNA, and is very sensitive to changes in exercise level. Physical activity acutely induces PGC-1α, and inactivity rapidly reduces its concentrations.

To meet increased mitochondrial oxygen demand, the oxygen supply needs to be augmented as well. Accordingly, muscles involved in exercise increase capillarity during endurance training. In this process, PGC-1α again plays a major role, as it is a major mediator for exercise-induced angiogenesis. In this regard, PGC-1α induces several angiogenic factors, such as vascular endothelial growth factor, platelet-derived growth factor, and angiopoietin-2.

To summarize, Ca^{2+} signaling and the AMPK system seem to be the major input determinants of the network contributing to endurance exercise adaptation, whereas ROS, hypoxia, and SIRT1 may serve to fine-tune the response. This signaling process is sensitive to substrate availability, in particular lipids for PPARs and glycogen for AMPK. All regulatory pathways converge on the transcriptional coactivator PGC-1α. PGC-1α binds and activates multiple transcription factors and nuclear receptors, can recruit chromatin remodeling complexes, and interacts with the splicing machinery coordinating transcriptional and posttranscriptional processes, the main consequences of which are an increase in the number and size of mitochondria and capillarity.

Strength Training

Strength training leads to muscle hypertrophy, with an increase in the muscle cross-sectional area. The increase in muscle volume/mass is fundamentally accounted for by an increase in myofibrils. This process is sensitive to sex hormone action. In particular, androgens interfere with multiple signaling pathways, stimulating cellular metabolism, enhancing growth, and inhibiting apoptosis. Androgen replacement is required in hypogonadal men for the increase in the number of myonuclei that underlies the hypertrophic effect induced by strength training [11].

The relative composition of muscles in terms of type I and type II fibers appears to be unchanged after strength exercise. However, after resistance training, there is a shift from subtype IIX to subtype IIA fibers. The regulation of muscle mass depends rather on modifications of muscle protein synthesis than on protein degradation. The synthesis rate of cell proteins in turn depends on both translational efficiency and translational capacity. In this regard, the mammalian target of rapamycin (mTOR) is considered the key factor integrating the multiple stimuli influencing accretion of myofibrillar proteins and muscle mass hypertrophy [12].

mTOR is a highly conserved serine/threonine kinase, which is a major regulatory protein for a number of cell processes, such as proliferation, growth, differentiation, protein synthesis, and substrate metabolism. mTOR has been established both as a component of the insulin cascade and an insulin-independent nutrient sensor. In particular, mTOR plays a key role in the regulation of muscle protein synthesis in response to exercise and nutrition, and in muscle intracellular signaling. This protein integrates inputs from insulin and growth factor signaling, amino acid availability, and energy status, leading to protein accumulation of the myofibrillar contractile apparatus.

In response to mechanical stimuli, muscles are capable of generating insulin-like growth factor (IGF)-1. IGF-1 stimulates its own receptor on the cell membrane, activating several intracellular signaling pathways, mainly the phosphatidylinositol 3-kinase (PI3K)-protein kinase B (or Akt)-mTOR pathway. This is considered the main pathway by which muscle protein synthesis is activated in response to growth factors. Akt proteins are a family of serine/threonine-specific kinases. Akt1 activation induces muscle hypertrophy through downstream signaling and is the dominant positive regulator of mTOR. It also inhibits the induction of atrophy signaling [13].

Interestingly, mechanical load per se appears to be sufficient to activate mTOR, and mTOR activation can occur in a PI3K-independent manner. The mechanoregulated signaling involved in muscle protein synthesis implies a cytoskeletal contribution, in which focal adhesion kinase has been shown to play a role. Furthermore, mechanical stimuli may enhance phospholipase D activity with increased intracellular levels of its product phosphatidic acid. This latter may also induce sustained activation of mTOR by a PIK3-AKT-independent pathway.

Combined Training
Interestingly, simultaneous strength and endurance training results in a reduced capacity to develop strength, whereas it did not compromise the ability to increase maximum oxygen uptake (VO_{2max}) [14]. It can thus be speculated that the AMPK-Akt master switch may predominate in the adaptive response to the combination of endurance and strength training. Interestingly, in this regard, although the mechanisms underlying these findings are still to be fully elucidated, AMPK and the protein regulated in the development and DNA damage responses (REDD1), which is a HIF-1 target gene and increases when there is hypoxic stress in the cell, suppress mTOR activity in skeletal muscles under low-energy/hypoxic conditions. Notably, REDD1 degradation is crucial for restoring mTOR signaling as cells recover from hypoxia.

Recent data showed that microRNAs (miRNA) may also have a role in the response to exercise training. miRNA are small noncoding RNAs, which may play a crucial role in RNA silencing in various regulatory networks. In particular, miRNA-696 has been shown to be involved in the regulation of PGC-1α, whereas miRNA-1 participates in the regulation of the IGF-1 transduction cascade.

Physiology of Energy Metabolism during Exercise

The mobilization of extracellular substrates is dependent upon the integration of the autonomic nervous and endocrine systems to coordinate an increase in both carbohydrate and fat availability. During the transition from rest to exercise, the sympathoadrenal system releases catecholamines and cortisol. Generally, during exercise, the arterial insulin level decreases and glucagon and growth hormone levels increase. The exercise-induced increase in catecholamine concentration is able to stimulate glycogen catabolism, to release glucose from the liver and to increase its availability in skeletal muscles, and triacylglycerol catabolism, to release nonesterified FA and glycerol from adipose tissue. The maintenance of blood glucose homeostasis during exercise represents a challenge because the rate of muscle glucose utilization increases severalfold, and intramuscular glycogen depots are rapidly consumed. During exercise, the rise in glucagon levels and the fall in insulin levels are both important for the increase in hepatic glucose production through gluconeogenesis, which is a key process in maintaining glucose release from the liver over time.

The increase in sympathetic nervous activity also greatly affects cardiovascular function, matching oxygen demand and substrate delivery to the contracting muscle whilst simultaneously making the maintenance of adequate blood pressure possible.

Substrate utilization, in terms of energy requirement, is a product of exercise intensity and duration. However, the relative contributions of these energy sources differ according to the characteristics of the exercise. The effects of exercise intensity on substrate utilization was elegantly studied by Romijn et al. [15], who employed a stable isotope methodology to determine the rates of carbohydrate and fat oxidation at exercise intensities that elicited 25, 65 and 85% of VO_{2max}. These authors showed that at 25% VO_{2max}, the primary contribution to energy turnover was through plasma nonesterified FA utilization, with a smaller contribution from plasma glucose oxidation. The metabolic response to exercise at 65% VO_{2max} resulted in an increase in the utilization of the intramuscular stores of glycogen or triglycerides. Interestingly, it was reported that at this intensity, the rate of fat oxidation was higher than either at 25 or 85% VO_{2max}. Conversely, the metabolic response to exercise at 85% VO_{2max} relied almost completely on carbohydrate utilization, whilst FA oxidation contributed less than 30% of the total energy turnover.

Regulation of Fat Utilization

At the onset of exercise, there is a large rise in the uptake and oxidation of long-chain FAs (LCFAs) in muscles, which increases up to 10-fold. Lipids used as energy in this condition originate from different sources: circulating albumin-bound LCFAs, circulating very-low-density lipoprotein triacylglycerols (TGs), FAs from TG stored in the muscle cell, and FAs liberated from adipose tissue. Lipolysis of TGs stored in adipose tissue is rapidly stimulated by the increase in catecholamines induced by exercise. There are multiple regulatory sites for LCFA utilization during exercise: (i) LCFA delivery from plasma and intramuscular TGs in lipid droplets; (ii) lipoprotein lipase activity, controlling delivery of LCFAs generated from circulating triglyceride-rich lipoproteins; (iii) LCFA transport across the plasma membrane; (iv) cytoplasmic handling of LCFAs, and (v) regulation within the mitochondria.

The importance of LCFA transport across the plasma membrane in skeletal muscles has been highlighted in several studies. The 88-kDa FA translocase/cluster of differentiation 36 (FAT/CD36) is a FA binding protein located at the plasma membrane, which acts as a regulator of FA transmembrane transport. Recent studies have suggested a role for FAT/CD36 in the acute increase in FA uptake in skeletal muscles seen in the transition from rest to exercise [16]. Interestingly, it has been found that, when exercise intensity increased to higher levels, FA uptake was still elevated compared to basal levels, despite FA oxidation being decreased to resting values. This finding supports the notion that muscle FA oxidation is mainly limited by factors inside the cell rather than by transmembrane transport.

Once LCFAs have entered the cell, they are converted to LCFA-CoA by long-chain acyl CoA synthetase. An efficient esterification maintains a low intracellular LCFA concentration and contributes to the uptake of LCFA. LCFA-CoA is subsequently transported across the mitochondrial membrane for final β-oxidation and generation of acetyl CoA. Regulation of the LCFA-CoA flow into mitochondria results from the fact that LCFAs have to be converted into their acylcarnitine derivatives in order to pass the mitochondrial inner membrane. This reaction is catalyzed by the enzyme carnitine palmitoyltransferase 1 (CPT1). Malonyl CoA is a potent inhibitor of CPT1. However, in human skeletal muscles, the decrease in malonyl CoA concentration from rest to exercise contributes to the increase in lipid oxidation at the onset of exercise, but plays a minor role in the regulation of lipid oxidation during sustained exercise.

Carnitine is a substrate for CTP1 and is required for the transport of activated LCFA-CoA across the mitochondrial membrane, being, therefore, essential for β-oxidation. It has been proposed that carnitine could act also as an acceptor of acetyl groups from acetyl CoA, by forming acetyl carnitine, when the rate of acetyl CoA synthesis from glycolysis, at high intensities of exercise, is in excess of its utilization by the Krebs cycle. It has been demonstrated that the concentration of acetyl carnitine within muscles is enhanced following increased exercise intensity. This phenomenon decreases the availability of free carnitine, resulting in low CPT1 activity and diminished supply of LCFA-CoA to β-oxidation. Hence, carnitine rather than malonyl-CoA seems to be a likely candidate in fine-tuning fat oxidation during exercise in humans [17].

Regulation of Glucose Utilization

Muscle glucose uptake is closely regulated by hormonal and nonhormonal mechanisms. During exercise, the rate of glucose uptake increases severalfold. Glucose uptake by contracting skeletal muscles is facilitated by diffusion, made possible by the presence of GLUT4 in the plasma membrane and an inward diffusion gradient for glucose.

There are three main sites of glucose utilization that can be regulated: (1) glucose delivery, (2) glucose transport, and (3) glucose metabolism.

Glucose uptake in vivo may be measured by the product of blood flow and arterio-venous glucose difference. The increase in blood flow is the component which mainly contributes to the exercise-induced increase in muscle glucose uptake. Skeletal muscle blood flow can increase up to 20 times from rest to high-intensity exercise. In addition to the increased blood flow to the contracting skeletal muscle during exercise, there is also the recruitment of capillaries, which increases the vessel surface area available for glucose delivery and exchange.

The increase in transmembrane glucose transport during exercise in skeletal muscles is due to the translocation of GLUT4 glucose carriers from intracellular sites to the sarcolemma. Interestingly, GLUT4 recruited by muscle contraction derives from a pool that is distinct from the GLUT4 pool disposed by insulin stimulation [18]. In addition, contraction seems to stimulate GLUT4 translocation through molecular mechanisms distinct from that of insulin. Nevertheless, these pathways converge, and a number of signaling molecules are involved in GLUT4 translocation activated by both insulin and muscle contraction [19].

During exercise, docking and fusion of the GLUT4 vesicles located in the intracellular storage sites seem to require complex interactions between proteins known as SNARE proteins (soluble N-ethylmaleimide-sensitive factor-attachment protein receptors) and regulatory proteins. In addition to the SNARE proteins, the actin cytoskeleton has been shown to play an important role in GLUT4 translocation.

Moreover, upstream signaling pathways that ultimately lead to GLUT4 translocation may include the activation of the cellular energy sensor AMPK, nitric oxide synthase and the calcium/calmodulin-dependent protein kinase kinases.

When the cell senses low energy (decreased ATP), AMPK appears to switch off ATP-consuming pathways and switch on alternative pathways for ATP regeneration. Physiological activation of AMPK occurs in working skeletal muscles in response to an AMP/ADP increase and an ATP decrease [20]. The hypothesis that AMPK may have a major role in contraction-stimulated increases in muscle glucose transport derives primarily from studies using 5-aminoimidazole-4-carboxamide ribonucleoside (AICAR), a compound that is taken up into skeletal muscles and metabolized by adenosine kinase to form a monophosphorylated derivative that mimics the effects of AMP on AMPK. Activation of AMPK by AICAR in resting muscles results in increased glucose uptake in muscles, and this effect is lost when either the catalytic or regulatory AMPK subunits are deficient.

Recent developments have revealed converging signaling pathways between contraction and insulin action in skeletal muscles. Such convergence points are GTPase-activating proteins of the TBC1 domain family (TBC1D1 and TBC1D4). In skeletal muscles, these proteins are targeted by both Akt and other kinases, including AMPK. The pathway linking TBC1D1 and TBC1D4 with GLUT4 translocation is thought to involve Rab (ras homologous from brain) proteins. These Rab proteins are involved in many membrane trafficking events, and active Rab proteins may recruit various effectors involved in vesicle budding, binding, and fusion. These interactions between insulin and contraction pathways may explain the additive effects of these stimuli on glucose transport and the benefits of exercise on skeletal muscle insulin action.

Once glucose has been transported across the sarcolemma, it is phosphorylated to glucose 6-phosphate in a reaction catalyzed by hexokinase II (HKII). Exercise is associated with a robust increase in HKII expression. Glucose phosphorylation is the first step in the metabolism of glucose through either the glycolytic and the oxidative pathways (responsible for energy production during exercise) or the glycogen synthesis after exercise. Glucose phosphorylation is another site of regulation for skeletal muscle glucose utilization. Studies in transgenic mice showed that during exercise, HKII overexpression led to increased glucose uptake at both normal and increased levels of GLUT4 expression. Conversely, GLUT4 overexpression itself did not lead to increased glucose uptake [21], indicating that, in the absence of HKII overexpression, it has little effect on muscle glucose utilization. These data suggest that the ability to phosphorylate glucose might be the rate-limiting step in glucose metabolism during exercise.

Metabolic Adaptations to Exercise Training in Skeletal Muscles

With aerobic training, the number of capillaries around each muscle fiber may increase by 20–30%. The phenomenon favors the exchange of gases and nutrients between the blood and the active muscle. Another change that occurs with aerobic training is a shift in muscle fiber type that favors substrate oxidation (from type IIb to IIa and I). After aerobic training, there is also an increase in the number and size of mitochondria. As a consequence, a trained muscle has an increased capacity to oxidize FAs. Other metabolic adaptations include an increase in carnitine transferase, which facilitates FA transport across the mitochondrial membrane, and in enzymes responsible for β-oxidation of LCFAs [22].

Exercise training enhances insulin sensitivity and induces increased expression of several key proteins involved in insulin-stimulated glucose metabolism, such as the glucose transporter GLUT4, HKII, and glycogen synthase.

Studies comparing individuals before and after training have demonstrated a reduced respiratory exchange ratio at the same relative workload. This indicates reduced carbohydrate and increased FA oxidation. Most available data show that, for the same absolute workload, trained individuals will have a slower rate of decline in both muscles and liver glycogen, which will also result in a reduced rate of decline in blood glucose. The slower utilization of muscle glycogen and blood glucose during exercise may be an important mechanism by which exercise training enhances endurance, since the depletion of carbohydrate stores and the development of hypoglycemia are related to the development of fatigue. In this context, it seems likely that the major beneficial effect of the adaptive increase in GLUT4 might be the increased ability to rapidly resynthesize glycogen to replenish muscle glycogen stores.

Alterations in Energy Metabolism during Exercise in Individuals with Insulin Resistance and Type 2 Diabetes

As discussed above, exercise and insulin share their metabolic effects on glucose handling. However, these effects recognize specific and distinct pathways, at least in part. Interestingly, although individuals with type 2 diabetes are typically insulin resistant, they are not resistant to the stimulatory effects of exercise on glucose uptake. Exercise may thus be helpful in reducing blood glucose levels and is considered a key element in the management of type 2 diabetes [23]. As regards the type of exercise, both aerobic and resistance training increase GLUT4 abundance and muscle glucose uptake, even in the presence of insulin resistance [24].

In subjects without diabetes, blood glucose shows little change during a single bout of moderate aerobic exercise, because glucose release from the liver matches the increase in skeletal muscle glucose uptake. Conversely, as exercise begins, glucose tends generally to decrease in subjects with type 2 diabetes, especially after submaximal aerobic training, because the utilization of blood glucose by skeletal muscles rises more than hepatic glucose production. However, during high-intensity exercise, plasma catecholamine levels may increase markedly, causing a striking rise in glucose production, which may even surpass the increase in glucose utilization. In subjects with type 2 diabetes, hyperglycemia may thus result from high-intensity exercise, especially in untrained patients, and may be observed up to a few hours after conclusion of exercise.

Some data suggest that a single bout of moderate-intensity aerobic training could be better in increasing muscle glucose uptake than a bout of resistance training of similar intensity and duration [25]. However, information is still limited, and we cannot exclude that differences might be rather due to different calorie expenditure of the exercise sessions than the type of exercise itself.

Notably, due to the synergistic effect of insulin and exercise, people with type 2 diabetes on treatment with insulin or insulin secretagogues, especially those taking sulfonylureas or glinides, may have an increased risk of hypoglycemia during exercise and for several hours after physical activity. This may require adaptation of antidiabetic therapy during exercise training sessions.

Chronic Effect of Exercise in Individuals with Type 2 Diabetes

Besides the acute, insulin-like but insulin-independent, effects of exercise, regular long-term aerobic training improves insulin sensitivity [26] by increasing the expression and/or activity of several proteins regulated by insulin and involved in fuel disposal. The training status influences both lipid and carbohydrate handling during physical activity. Importantly, regular exercise may improve fat storage and fat oxidation capacity in muscles particularly in insulin-resistant obese and type 2 diabetic subjects.

An increase in capillary density is also observed in response to aerobic exercise training, both in healthy and insulin-resistant individuals. This phenomenon facilitates the diffusion of glucose from the capillaries into the muscle cells, particularly in subjects with type 2 diabetes.

Strength training, as well, appears to improve insulin action and may be combined with aerobic training in subjects with type 2 diabetes. The favorable effect of strength training may be in part due to skeletal muscle hypertrophy, which increases the mass of tissue responsive to insulin in terms of glucose storage and utilization. However, strength exercise may also improve insulin action by stimulating the expression and/or activity of insulin receptors, glucose transporters, and several enzymes involved in glucose metabolism. The differences in the mechanisms underlying the enhancement of insulin action obtained by aerobic and resistance training are still partially unclear. However, there is evidence that, in individuals with type 2 diabetes, structured combined physical training may be associated with HbA1c reduction which is greater than with aerobic or strength training alone. In this regard, the American Diabetes Association and the American College of Sports Medicine have stated that a combination of aerobic and resistance exercise training is recommended to improve glucose control in subjects with type 2 diabetes [23]. However, it should be remembered that for weight loss/maintenance, in obese diabetic individuals, a greater exercise volume may be required, and the most successful plan is a combination of diet, exercise, and behavioral modifications.

Exercise and Metabolic Inflexibility
Whereas skeletal muscles utilize both carbohydrate and FAs at rest and during contractions, the extent to which it relies on these energy sources depends on several issues, such as substrate availability, metabolic demand, capacity of transport, and substrate utilization. Interestingly, in subjects with insulin resistance, there is metabolic inflexibility [27], i.e. reduced ability of tissues to adapt their metabolism to changes in physiological conditions. This abnormality may be linked to the etiology of obesity, type 2 diabetes, and other conditions characterized by alterations in insulin action. Generally, metabolic inflexibility is seen as the impairment in the capacity of tissues to shift from lipid to glucose oxidation when passing from low-insulin fasting conditions to high-insulin glucose-stimulated conditions. Similar abnormalities could occur when passing from resting to exercise conditions, but there have been few investigations into this phenomenon. During acute exercise, with an increase in exercise intensity, there is a physiological shift from predominantly fat to almost total glucose oxidation. Limited data suggest that obese subjects with type 2 diabetes may have a reduced capacity to rely on FAs during moderate-intensity aerobic exercise [28]. However, the results are controversial. Further research is needed in this field.

Alterations in FA availability, uptake, and oxidation are potentially key factors in metabolic inflexibility and insulin resistance. Interestingly, the capacity for fat oxidation is positively related to the training status and body leanness. During fasting conditions, obese individuals show a reduced capacity for FA oxidation compared with normal-weight subjects, whereas during insulin-stimulated conditions they have an impaired ability to increase glucose oxidation. In obese, insulin-resistant individuals, diet-induced weight loss improves insulin-stimulated glucose utilization, but does not seem to be able to alter fasting fat oxidation. However, interestingly, in these individuals, regular aerobic training may increase both lipid oxidation during fasting conditions and glucose oxidation during insulin-stimulated conditions [29]. This suggests that physical inactivity may be relevant in the impaired fat oxidation of obesity, further supporting the importance of adding exercise training to diet-based weight loss programs in obese people.

References

1 Plowman SA, Smith DL: Exercise Physiology for Health, Fitness, and Performance, ed 4. Philadelphia, Wolters Kluwer Health/Lippincott Williams & Wilkins, 2014.

2 Tiidus PM, Russell Tupling A, Houston ME: Biochemistry Primer for Exercise Science, ed 4. Champaign, Human Kinetics, 2012.

3 Mougios V: Exercise Biochemistry. Champaign, Human Kinetics, 2006.

4 McArdle WD, Katch FI, Katch VL: Exercise Physiology: Energy, Nutrition, and Human Performance, ed 6. Philadelphia, Lippincott Williams & Wilkins, 2007.

5 Stryer L: Biochemistry. New York, Freeman, 1995.

6 Baldwin KM, Haddad F: Effects of different activity and inactivity paradigms on myosin heavy chain gene expression in striated muscle. J Appl Physiol (1985) 2001;90:345–357.

7 Prior BM, Yang HT, Terjung RL: What makes vessels grow with exercise training? J Appl Physiol (1985) 2004;97:1119–1128.
8 Narci MV, Hoppeler H, Kayser B, Landoni L, Claassen H, Gavardi C, Conti M, Cerretelli P: Human quadriceps cross-sectional area, torque and neural activation during 6 months strength training. Acta Physiol Scand 1996;157:175–186.
9 Hardie DG, Sakamoto K: AMPK: a key sensor of fuel and energy status in skeletal muscle. Physiology (Bethesda) 2006;21:48–60.
10 Spiegelmann BM: Transcriptional control of energy homeostasis through the PGC1 coactivators. Novartis Found Symp 2007;286:3–6.
11 Kvorning T, Kadi F, Schjerling P, Andersen M, Brixen K, Suetta C, Madsen K: The activity of satellite cells and myonuclei following 8 weeks of strength training in young men with suppressed testosterone levels. Acta Physiol (Oxf) 2015;213:676–687.
12 Kimball SR, Jefferson LS: Control of translation initiation through integration of signals generated by hormones, nutrients, and exercise. J Biol Chem 2010;285:29027–29032.
13 Cleasby ME, Reinten TA, Cooney GJ, James DE, Kraegen EW: Functional studies of Akt isoform specificity in skeletal muscle in vivo; maintained insulin sensitivity despite reduced insulin receptor substrate-1 expression. Mol Endocrinol 2007;21:215–228.
14 Nader GA: Concurrent strength and endurance training: from molecules to man. Med Sci Sports Exerc 2006;38:1965–1970.
15 Romijn JA, Coyle EF, Sidossis LS, Gastaldelli A, Horowitz JA, Endert E, Wolfe RR: Regulation of endogenous fat and carbohydrate metabolism in relation to exercise intensity and duration. Am J Physiol Endocrinol Metab 1993;265:E380–E391.
16 Jeppensen J, Albers PH, Rose AJ, Birk JB, Schjerling P, Dzamko N, Steimberg GR, Kiens B: Contraction-induced skeletal muscle FAT/CD36 trafficking and FA uptake is AMPK independent. J Lipid Res 2011;52:699–711.
17 Van Loon LJ, Greenhaff PL, Constantin-Teodosiu D, Saris WH, Wagenmakers AJ: The effects of increasing exercise intensity on muscle fuel utilization in humans. J Physiol 2001;536:295–304.
18 Coderre L, Kandror KV, Vallega G, Pilch PF: Identification and characterization of an exercise-sensitive pool of glucose transporters in skeletal muscle. J Biol Chem 1995;270:27584–27588.
19 Kramer HF, Witczak CA, Taylor EB, Fujii N, Hirshman MF, Goodyear LJ: AS160 regulates insulin- and contraction-stimulated glucose uptake in mouse skeletal muscle. J Biol Chem 2006;281:31478–31485.
20 Wojtaszewski JFP, Nielsen P, Hansen BF, Richter EA, Kiens B: Isoform-specific and exercise intensity-dependent activation of 5′-AMP-activated protein kinase in human skeletal muscle. J Physiol 2000;528:221–226.
21 Wasserman DH: Four grams of glucose. Am J Physiol Endocrinol Metab 2009;296:E11–E21.
22 Mittendorfer B, Klein S: Physiological factors that regulate the use of endogenous fat and carbohydrate fuels during endurance exercise. Nutr Res Rev 2003;16:97–108.
23 Colberg SR, Sigal RJ, Fernhall B, Regensteiner JG, Blissmer BJ, Rubin RR, Chasan-Taber L, Albright AL, Braun B: Exercise and type 2 diabetes: the American College of Sports Medicine and the American Diabetes Association: joint position statement. Diabetes Care 2010;33:e147–e167.
24 Christ-Roberts CY, Pratipanawatr T, Pratipanawatr W, Berria R, Belfort R, Kashyap S, Mandarino LJ: Exercise training increases glycogen synthase activity and GLUT4 expression but not insulin signaling in overweight nondiabetic and type 2 diabetic subjects. Metabolism 2004;53:1233–1242.
25 Bacchi E, Negri C, Trombetta M, Zanolin ME, Lanza M, Bonora E, Moghetti P: Differences in the acute effects of aerobic and resistance exercise in subjects with type 2 diabetes: results from the RAED2 Randomized Trial. PLoS One 2012;7:e49937.
26 Bacchi E, Negri C, Zanolin ME, Milanese C, Faccioli N, Trombetta M, Zoppini G, Cevese A, Bonadonna RC, Schena F, Bonora E, Lanza M, Moghetti P: Metabolic effects of aerobic training and resistance training in type 2 diabetic subjects: a randomized controlled trial (the RAED2 study). Diabetes Care 2012;35:676–682.
27 Storlien L, Oakes ND, Kelley DE: Metabolic flexibility. Proc Nutr Soc 2004;63:363–368.
28 Ghanassia E, Brun JF, Fedou C, Raynaud E, Mercier J: Substrate oxidation during exercise: type 2 diabetes is associated with a decrease in lipid oxidation and an earlier shift towards carbohydrate utilization. Diabetes Metab 2006;32:604–610.
29 Goodpaster BH, Wolfe RR, Kelley DE: Effects of obesity on substrate utilization during exercise. Obes Res 2002;10:575–584.

Prof. Paolo Moghetti
Division of Endocrinology, Diabetes and Metabolism
Department of Medicine, University of Verona
Piazzale Stefani 1, IT–37126 Verona (Italy)
E-Mail paolo.moghetti@univr.it

Lanfranco F, Strasburger CJ (eds): Sports Endocrinology.
Front Horm Res. Basel, Karger, 2016, vol 47, pp 58–67 (DOI: 10.1159/000445157)

Endocrine Responses to Exercise in the Developing Child and Adolescent

Erick Richmond[a] · Alan D. Rogol[b]

[a]Pediatric Endocrinology, National Children's Hospital, San José, Costa Rica; [b]Pediatric Endocrinology, University of Virginia, Charlottesville, Va., USA

Abstract

The impact of exercise training on the neuroendocrine control of the pituitary in the developing child is complex and the exact mechanisms are not fully understood. Multiple determinants influence adaptive hypothalamic-pituitary secretory responses to physical stress, namely, training intensity and duration, nutrition and energy balance, gender, age, sex, and sexual maturation status. The increase in growth hormone (GH) in response to acute exercise is dependent on pubertal status; children in more advanced pubertal stages respond with larger peak GH concentrations compared to those in earlier stages. The adolescent female athlete is more prone to menstrual disorders than the more mature athlete, and recent data suggest that athletes may be able to reverse menstrual disorders by increasing their dietary energy intake without decreasing their exercise levels. The thyroid changes observed are of minor impact, practically reflecting the relative negative energy balance during strenuous exercise. Studies that evaluated changes in cortisol secretion during aerobic exercise in children and adolescents show either an increase or no change in response to the exercise bout. Recent research showed that physical activity is an important contributor to bone strength prior to adolescence and increasing levels of physical activity during childhood likely enhance optimal bone strength.

Physical activity plays a key role in tissue growth and anabolism in the developing child. Exercise stimulates somatic growth and muscle development, strengthens bones, and contributes to the development of the cardiovascular, respiratory, and thermoregulatory systems. The impact of exercise training on the neuroendocrine control of the pituitary is complex. Multiple determinants influence adaptive hypothalamic-pituitary secretory responses to physical stress, namely, training intensity and duration, nutrition and energy balance, gender, age, sex, and sexual maturation status. Most of the research done evaluating hormonal changes related to exercise is focused on the adult population, only a few studies include children and adolescents.

The aim of this paper is to summarize the best evidence of endocrine responses to exercise in the developing child.

Growth Hormone-Insulin-Like Growth Factor-1 Axis

The growth hormone (GH)-insulin-like growth factor (IGF)-1 axis is composed of hormones, growth factors, binding proteins, and receptors that regulate essential life processes such as growth and maturation.

IGF-1 is synthesized and released from multiple tissues. However, most of the circulating IGF-1 is produced by the liver, where the expression of the IGF-1 gene is regulated by GH [1]. In addition to classical endocrine effects exerted by circulating IGFs, locally produced IGFs exert paracrine as well as autocrine effects on cell proliferation. The serum levels of IGF-1 are much greater than those of almost any other growth factor or peptide hormone. However, less than 1% of the circulating IGF-1 is present in the free (active) form, and the rest is bound to binding proteins [2].

Physical activity plays a pivotal role in tissue growth and anabolism in the developing child, but the exact mechanisms are not fully understood. The combination of rapid growth, high levels of physical activity, and increases in GH, IGF-1, and sex steroid levels suggests the possibility of integrated mechanisms linking exercise with anabolic responses.

Exercise-induced increase in IGF-1, one of the most important anabolic factors, occurs within minutes after the onset of supramaximal exercise [3]. It is believed that the increase in IGF-1 plays a key role in exercise training-induced muscle hypertrophy. Most of the current knowledge regarding the importance of the GH response to exercise is based on studies of the effect of aerobic-type exercise [4]. The increase in GH in response to acute exercise is dependent on pubertal status: children in more advanced pubertal stages respond with larger peak GH concentrations compared to those in earlier stages, perhaps related to the increase in sex steroids [5].

Among other determinants of neuroendocrine responses to exercise training is the acuteness versus chronicity of the training or exercise stimulus. Acute exercise induces a variety of short-term hormonal changes, including the nearly immediate secretion of GH, whereas the result of chronic training is not necessarily identical [6]. In terms of resistance exercise, many factors influence the magnitude of the response of GH, including the muscle mass, the training intensity, the rest period in between sets, the total volume, and the workload. In addition, the change in GH is closely related to the increase in lactate, which reflects the effect of all factors previously presented [6].

With the increased participation in competitive sports at a young age, a major concern is the possibility that inadequate and/or excessive exercise training during childhood might stunt growth, because of a negative influence on the GH-IGF-1 axis and also due to a possible negative caloric balance [7]. In an early study in prepubertal female gymnasts, IGF-1 was measured at baseline and over 3 days of intensive training lasting 3.5–5.5 h. Concentrations of IGF-1 decreased by 25% after the 3 days of training with no concurrent changes in GH levels [8]. In a follow-up study, adolescent girls went through a 5-week endurance training period with no caloric restriction, and a decrease in IGF-1 levels was observed in the intervention but not in the control group [9]. A study of the GH-IGF-1 axis in undernourished adolescent wrestlers showed increases in GH concentrations and concomitant decreases in IGF-1 concentrations during the competitive season, but all hormone levels returned to normal ranges after the competitive season [10].

Recent studies document that percent body fat, in particular visceral fat (intra-abdominal) accumulation, negatively influences pulsatile GH secretion by suppressing the mass of GH secreted per burst and shortening the half-life of GH in the circulation [11], and excess adiposity negatively affects IGF-1 concentrations [12]. Some evidence suggests that in children as in adults, high levels of body fat may blunt the catecholamine response to acute exercise. A well-designed study demonstrated a blunted catecholamine release in response to a 30-min, high-intensity, intermittent cycling bout in obese children versus lean participants. The authors suggested that the blunted adrenergic response could be linked to a blunted GH release in obese children [4]. A recent study showed that the blunting of the GH response to exercise was dependent on the degree of obesity: the more obese the children, the larger the blunting of the GH response [13].

Hypothalamic-Pituitary-Gonadal Axis

The response of estradiol and testosterone to exercise in children has been evaluated in a few studies. During childhood, both boys and girls have similar blood concentrations of testosterone; however, during mid-puberty, levels of testosterone increase in a robust manner in boys. Testosterone enhances muscle hypertrophy, strength, endurance, and power [14]. Exercise-induced sex hormone responses at different stages of sexual maturation were tested in a 3-year longitudinal experiment on 34 girls aged 11–12 years. Estradiol and testosterone responses were highest in Tanner stage V [5]. In adolescent males aged 16–17 years, a higher testosterone response to a graded exercise protocol has been shown when the subjects were in Tanner stage V versus Tanner stage IV of genital development [15]. A 32% increase in testosterone concentrations was demonstrated in a study of junior elite weight lifters aged 16–18 years after a traditional weight lifting session involving high-intensity, high-speed resistance training exercises [16]. Resistance exercise in adolescents and young male adult athletes resulted in a lower increase in testosterone concentrations in the younger males [17]. Acute testosterone responses in male junior triathletes (15.8 ± 1.8 years) after

16 training sessions were evaluated within a 2-week period in a recent study. After the training sessions, testosterone concentrations were significantly higher at all time points during the last compared to first training session [18].

More studies on the testosterone response to exercise in young children and girls are needed. From the scant information available, it is suggested that there is an acute increase in testosterone concentrations after resistance exercise in adolescent boys, but the magnitude of the increment is lower when compared with young adult males.

Age at menarche is influenced by intense exercise training. Although genetic factors also have a strong influence on menarcheal age, dancers and gymnasts have delayed menarche compared with their sedentary sisters even though they are genetically very similar [19]. Puberty involves maturation of axillary and pubic hair as well as breast development. Interestingly, when young athletes are forced (often because of injury) to interrupt their gymnastics or dance training, rapid progression of Tanner breast stages may occur [20]. The pubertal maturation of the breast is primarily dependent on ovarian hormones, with little or no influence of adrenal steroids. By contrast, pubic hair maturation can proceed with normal adolescent increases in adrenal androgen secretion, without significant increases in ovarian hormones. The discrepancy in the degree of breast development compared with pubic hair maturation through the Tanner stages may be a clue to hypothalamic adaptive changes related to exercise training and/or other stressors. It has been reported that pubic hair development occurred at a normal age in young woman dancers, yet breast development and age at menarche tended to be delayed [21].

The development of amenorrhea with exercise training has been attributed to many factors, but the leading candidates are: (1) decreased energy availability owing to greater energy expenditure of exercise than dietary energy intake or (2) abnormal levels of stress hormones owing to chronic stress of exercise. In support to the first theory, it has recently been demonstrated that short-term induction of menstrual cycle changes with exercise can be prevented by adequate dietary compensation, and the authors suggested that athletes may be able to reverse menstrual disorders by increasing their dietary energy intake without decreasing their exercise levels [22].

A well-designed study in sedentary young women demonstrated that the dependence of LH pulsatility and ovarian function on energy availability declines with gynecological age, which partially explains the common observation that the adolescent female athlete is more prone to menstrual disorders than the more mature athlete [23].

Thyroid Axis

Thyroid hormones are important regulators of energy metabolism and may influence energy processes during physical exercise. There are controversial results concerning thyroid hormone metabolism during strenuous exercise in adult athletes and only scant data exist concerning the impact of strenuous exercise on thyroid hormone metabolism in children and adolescents. Although some studies demonstrate a transient change in thyroid hormones during intense physical performance, most studies agree that these changes are of minor impact, practically reflecting the relative negative energy balance during strenuous exercise. This state of hypometabolism during intense physical performance has also been confirmed in highly trained female young athletes.

Young male monozygotic twins were investigated after a 93-day training period while their energy intake remained at the level before training. Their resting metabolic rate decreased by 8% after training, while their plasma levels of T_3, free T_3, and T_4 were also reduced after training. The authors concluded that exercise training associated with a substantial negative energy balance may induce a transient decrease in thyroid hormone concentrations [24].

Another study documenting thyroid hormone levels during a 3-week professional road cycling competition demonstrated that although TSH and total T_3 levels remained stable before and during the 3 weeks of cycling, there was a significant increase in free T_4, free T_3, and T_4 levels in the 3rd week of competition [25].

Girls practicing intensive physical exercise have shown a low T_3/T_4 ratio; this reduction in T_3 levels, combined with a reduction in IGF-1 levels, has been related with the hypometabolic state of intensive physical exercise during childhood and adolescence while indicating the importance of adequate nutrition in highly trained young athletes [26].

Adrenal Axis

The hypothalamic-pituitary-adrenal axis consists of three structurally independent components including the hypothalamus, the anterior pituitary, and the adrenal cortex. These structures intimately interact through the release of neuroendocrine messengers. In response to physiological or psychological stress, the anterior pituitary releases adrenocorticotropic hormone that stimulates the release of cortisol from the adrenal gland. Most studies that evaluated changes in cortisol secretion during aerobic exercise in children and adolescents show either an increase or no change in response to the exercise bout. Investigations that showed an increase in cortisol secretion include a recent study aimed to determine the effects of a single high-intensity interval training session on salivary cortisol levels in trained boys and men. Twenty-three boys 10–12 years of age and 25 men 25–35 years of age performed 4 consecutive high-intensity interval training sessions. Salivary cortisol in boys and men increased from 5.55 ± 3.3 to 15.13 ± 9.7 nmol/l (+173%) and from 7.07 ± 4.7 to 19.19 ± 12.7 nmol/l (+171%), respectively [27]. In another study in 10-year-old male children, cortisol concentrations were increased by 43 and 57% after 15 and 30 min of intense exercise compared to resting conditions, respectively, and even remained elevated after a 15-min recovery from exercise [28]. A longitudinal exercise study demonstrated that the cortisol response to acute exercise was the highest during mid-puberty (Tanner stages II and III) in comparison with late puberty (Tanner stages IV and V) [5]. A more recent study evaluated cortisol responses to incremental-stage exercises to exhaustion in adolescents (Tanner stages IV and V) and young adults. Cortisol responses of the adolescents at Tanner stages IV and V as well as those of the adults progressively increased from rest to the end of the exercise test at the final sprint. However, no group differences occurred in the magnitude of responses between the adolescents (Tanner stages IV and V) and the adults. There was a slight tendency for cortisol levels of adolescents to be elevated at rest in comparison to the young adults. [15].

The response of cortisol to exercise is highly variable. Most studies that showed no response of cortisol to exercise included intermittent exercise protocols and were performed in the morning. It is possible that cortisol concentrations were in their morning peak and then decreased following the natural circadian rhythm. If this is the case, the exercise-induced rise in cortisol might be masked by the morning's peak level.

Studies that showed no change in circulating cortisol concentrations in response to exercise include two studies that used an intermittent-intense cycling bout with ten 2-min exercise intervals separated by 1 min of rest. Both studies included children with a wide age range and showed that cortisol concentrations were lower in the recovery period 1 h after exercise compared to concentrations at baseline and immediately after exercise [4, 29]. Salivary cortisol measurements in adolescent female tennis players after 16 weeks of training also showed a low overall output of salivary cortisol and a blunted response to awakening [30].

Bone

Positive effects of exercise on bone, including increased bone mineral density, have been demonstrated in several studies. Increasing physical activity levels throughout the lifespan is a general recommendation for preventing the development of osteoporosis.

Physical activity seems to be an important contributor to bone strength prior to adolescence, and increasing levels of physical activity during childhood likely enhance optimal bone strength. The Iowa Bone Development Study showed that for boys and girls, moderate and vigorous physical activity was a positive independent predictor of femoral neck bone strength [31]. Relatively 'little' exercise is necessary to induce a positive impact on bone density in children. A 7-month jumping intervention (10 min, 3 times per week) in prepubertal boys showed a significant bone mineral accrual at several bone regions [32]. A smaller study in Sweden also described that daily vigorous physical activity for at least 25 min seems to improve femoral neck bone strength in children [33]. In a population-based, 6-year, controlled exercise intervention study in children 6–9 years of age, daily physical exercise improved bone mass and bone size in girls, and bone mass in boys, without affecting the fracture risk [34]. A large study in the United Kingdom evaluated 1,748 boys and girls (mean age 15.5 years), and investigators found that vigorous day-to-day physical activity is associated with indices of cortical bone mass and geometry in adolescents, whereas light or moderate physical activity has no detectable association. The authors suggested that promoting physical activity in childhood is unlikely to benefit skeletal development unless high-impact activities are also increased [35]. A study in Canada analyzed adult bone geometry, volumetric density, and estimated strength in retired gymnasts compared to controls 10 years after retirement from sports. Former female gymnasts have significantly better geometric and densitometric properties, as well as estimated strength, at the radius and tibia 10 years after retirement compared to females who did not participate in gymnastics in childhood and adolescence [36]. The age when training starts is important. A study in female tennis and squash players showed that the benefit of playing to forearm and arm bone mass is about two times greater if females start playing at or before menarche rather than after it [37].

It has become evident, however, that too much exercise in combination with deficient energy intake may be detrimental to bone in some individuals. Intense training in some female athletes may lead to the development of amenorrhea and a corresponding decrease in bone mineral content [38]. Amenorrheic athletes have been able to reverse menstrual disorders and increase bone mass by reducing training volume and improving nutrition [39].

Calcium-regulating hormones play an important role in bone metabolism. It is known that parathyroid hormone (PTH) stimulates both bone resorption and bone formation. The response of PTH to acute exercise bouts is quite variable within studies; very scarce data exist in children and adolescents. A study of high-school female athletes in Japan demonstrated that the amount of exercise affects PTH response, moderate exercise suppresses PTH secretion, while strenuous exercise induces continuous secretion, which has a negative effect on bone mineral density [40]. A more recent study in premenarcheal female rhythmic gymnasts, aged 9–13 years, showed a positive association of years of training with cortical bone mineral content, area, and thickness independent of chronological age. In this study, biochemical analysis revealed that rhythmic gymnasts had lower PTH levels compared with controls [41].

Further research is needed to determine the exact direction of changes in basal PTH levels in response to different training protocols and whether these changes can be considered beneficial or detrimental to bone.

Conclusion

In summary, research in recent years has made substantial progress in the field of exercise endocrinology, although most of the studies are done in young adult subjects. It is clear that the impact of exercise training on the neuroendocrine control of the pituitary in the developing child is complex. The increase in GH in response to acute exercise is dependent on pubertal status; children in more advanced pubertal stages respond with larger peak GH concentrations than those in earlier stages. The development of amenorrhea with exercise training may be caused by inadequate nutrition and/or abnormal levels of stress hormones, but recent studies suggest that athletes may be able to reverse menstrual disorders by increasing their dietary energy intake without decreasing their exercise levels. Only scant data exist concerning the impact of strenuous exercise on thyroid hormone metabolism in children and adolescents. Most studies agree that the thyroid changes observed are of minor impact, practically reflecting the relative negative energy balance during strenuous exercise. The response of cortisol to exercise is highly variable. Studies that evaluated changes in cortisol secretion during aerobic exercise in children and adolescents show either an increase or no change in response to the exercise bout. Recent research showed that physical activity is an important contributor to bone strength prior to adolescence, and increasing levels of physical activity during childhood likely enhance optimal bone strength.

References

1 Stewart CE, Rotwein P: Growth, differentiation, and survival: multiple physiological functions for insulin-like growth factors. Physiol Rev 1996;76:1005–1026.

2 Hizuka N, Takano K, Asakawa K, Sukegawa I, Fukuda I, Demura H, Iwashita M, Adachi T, Shizume K: Measurement of free form of insulin-like growth factor 1 in human plasma. Growth Regul 1991;1:51–55.

3 Kraemer WJ, Harman FS, Vos NH, Gordon SE, Nindl BC, Marx JO, Gómez AL, Volek JS, Ratamess NA, Mazzetti SA, Bush JA, Dohi K, Newton RU, Häkkinen K: Effects of exercise and alkalosis on serum insulin-like growth factor I and IGF-binding protein-3. Can J Appl Physiol 2000;25:127–138.

4 Eliakim A, Nemet D, Zaldivar F, McMurray RG, Culler FL, Galassetti P, Cooper DM: Reduced exercise-associated response of the GH-IGF-I axis and catecholamines in obese children and adolescents. J Appl Physiol 2006;100:1630–1637.

5 Viru A, Laaneots L, Karelson K, Smirnova T, Viru M: Exercise-induced hormone responses in girls at different stages of sexual maturation. Eur J Appl Physiol Occup Physiol 1998;77:401–408.

6 Kanaley JA, Weltman JY, Veldhuis JD, Rogol AD, Hartman ML, Weltman A: Human growth hormone response to repeated bouts of aerobic exercise. J Appl Physiol 1997;83:1756–1761.

7 Roemmich JN, Richmond EJ, Rogol AD: Consequences of sport training during puberty. J Endocrinol Invest 2001;24:708–715.

8 Jahreis G, Kauf E, Fröhner G, Schmidt HE: Influence of intensive exercise on insulin-like growth factor 1, thyroid and steroid hormones in female gymnasts. Growth Regul 1991;1:95–99.

9 Eliakim A, Brasel JA, Mohan S, Barstow TJ, Berman N, Cooper DM: Physical fitness, endurance training, and the growth hormone-insulin-like growth factor 1 system in adolescent females. J Clin Endocrinol Metab 1996;81:3986–3992.

10 Roemmich JN, Sinning WE: Weight loss and wrestling training: effects on growth-related hormones. J Appl Physiol 1997;82:1760–1764.

11 Iranmanesh A, Grisso B, Veldhuis JD: Low basal and persistent pulsatile growth hormone secretion are revealed in normal and hyposomatotropic men studied with a new ultrasensitive chemiluminescence assay. J Clin Endocrinol Metab 1994;78:526–535.

12 Rubin DA, Castner DM, Pham H, Ng J, Adams E, Judelson DA: Hormonal and metabolic responses to a resistance exercise protocol in lean children, obese children and lean adults. Pediatr Exerc Sci 2014;26:444–454.

13 Oliver SR, Rosa JS, Minh TD, Pontello AM, Flores RL, Barnett M, Galassetti PR: Dose-dependent relationship between severity of pediatric obesity and blunting of the growth hormone response to exercise. J Appl Physiol 2010;108:21–27.

14 Spiering BA, Kraemer WJ, Vingren JL, Ratamess NA, Anderson JM, Armstrong LE, Nindl BC, Volek JS, Häkkinen K, Maresh CM: Elevated endogenous testosterone concentrations potentiate muscle androgen receptor responses to resistance exercise. J Steroid Biochem Mol Biol 2009;114:195–199.
15 Hackney AC, Viru M, VanBruggen M, Janson T, Karelson K, Viru A: Comparison of the hormonal responses to exhaustive incremental exercise in adolescent and young adult males. Arq Bras Endocrinol Metabol 2011;55:213–218.
16 Kraemer WJ, Fry AC, Warren BJ, Stone MH, Fleck SJ, Kearney JT, Conroy BP, Maresh CM, Weseman CA, Triplett NT: Acute hormonal responses in elite junior weightlifters. Int J Sports Med 1992;13:103–109.
17 Pullinen T, Mero A, MacDonald E, Pakarinen A, Komi PV: Plasma catecholamine and serum testosterone responses to four units of resistance exercise in young and adult male athletes. Eur J Appl Physiol Occup Physiol 1998;77:413–420.
18 Zinner C, Wahl P, Achtzehn S, Reed JL, Mester J: Acute hormonal responses before and after 2 weeks of HIT in well trained junior triathletes. Int J Sports Med 2014;35:316–322.
19 Treloar SA, Martin NG: Age at menarche as a fitness trait: nonadditive genetic variance detected in a large twin sample. Am J Hum Genet 1990;47:137–148.
20 Frisch RE, Gotz-Welbergen AV, McArthur JW, Albright T, Witschi J, Bullen B, Birnholz J, Reed RB, Hermann H: Delayed menarche and amenorrhea of college athletes in relation to age of onset of training. JAMA 1981;246:1559–1563.
21 Warren MP: The effects of exercise on pubertal progression and reproductive function in girls. J Clin Endocrinol Metab 1980;51:1150–1157.
22 Loucks AB, Verdun M, Heath EM: Low energy availability, not stress of exercise, alters LH pulsatility in exercising women. J Appl Physiol 1998;84:37–46.
23 Loucks AB: The response of luteinizing hormone pulsatility to 5 days of low energy availability disappears by 14 years of gynecological age. J Clin Endocrinol Metab 2006;91:3158–3164.
24 Tremblay A, Poehlman ET, Despres JP, Theriault G, Danforth E, Bouchard C: Endurance training with constant energy intake in identical twins: changes over time in energy expenditure and related hormones. Metabolism 1997;46:499–503.
25 Chicharro JL, Hoyos J, Bandres F, Terrados N, Fernandez B, Lucia A: Thyroid hormone levels during a 3-week professional road cycling competition. Horm Res 2001;56:159–164.
26 Jahreis G, Kauf E, Fröhner G, Schmidt HE: Influence of intensive exercise on insulin-like growth factor 1, thyroid and steroid hormones in female gymnasts. Growth Regul 1991;1:95–99.
27 Engel F, Härtel S, Wagner MO, Strahler J, Bös K, Sperlich B: Hormonal, metabolic, and cardiorespiratory responses of young and adult athletes to a single session of high-intensity cycle exercise. Pediatr Exerc Sci 2014;26:485–494.
28 Del Corral P, Mahon AD, Duncan GE, Howe CA, Craig BW: The effect of exercise on serum and salivary cortisol in male children. Med Sci Sports Exerc 1994;26:1297–1301.
29 Galassetti PR, Iwanaga K, Crisostomo M, Zaldivar FP, Larson J, Pescatello A: Inflammatory cytokine, growth factor and counterregulatory responses to exercise in children with type 1 diabetes and healthy controls. Pediatr Diabetes 2006;7:16–24.
30 Filaire E, Ferreira JP, Oliveira M, Massart A: Diurnal patterns of salivary alpha-amylase and cortisol secretion in female adolescent tennis players after 16 weeks of training. Psychoneuroendocrinology 2013;38:1122–1132.
31 Janz KF, Gilmore JM, Levy SM, Letuchy EM, Burns TL, Beck TJ: Physical activity and femoral neck bone strength during childhood: the Iowa Bone Development Study. Bone 2007;41:216–222.
32 MacKelvie KJ, McKay HA, Petit MA, Moran O, Khan KM: Bone mineral response to a 7-month randomized controlled, school-based jumping intervention in 121 prepubertal boys: associations with ethnicity and body mass index. J Bone Miner Res 2002;17:834–844.
33 Sardinha LB, Baptista F, Ekelund U: Objectively measured physical activity and bone strength in 9-year-old boys and girls. Pediatrics 2008;122:728–736.
34 Detter F, Rosengren BE, Dencker M, Lorentzon M, Nilsson JA, Karlsson MK: A 6-year exercise program improves skeletal traits without affecting fracture risk: a prospective controlled study in 2,621 children. J Bone Miner Res 2014;29:1325–1336.
35 Sayers A, Mattocks C, Deere K, Ness A, Riddoch C, Tobias JH: Habitual levels of vigorous, but not moderate or light, physical activity is positively related to cortical bone mass in adolescents. J Clin Endocrinol Metab 2011;96:793–802.
36 Erlandson MC, Kontulainen SA, Chilibeck PD, Arnold CM, Faulkner RA, Baxter-Jones AD: Former premenarcheal gymnasts exhibit site-specific skeletal benefits in adulthood after long-term retirement. J Bone Miner Res 2012;27:2298–2305.
37 Kannus P, Haapasalo H, Sankelo M, Sievänen H, Pasanen M, Heinonen A, Oja P, Vuori I: Effect of starting age of physical activity on bone mass in the dominant arm of tennis and squash players. Ann Intern Med 1995;123:27–31.
38 Drinkwater BL, Nilson K, Chesnut CH, Bremner WJ, Shainholtz S, Southworth MB: Bone mineral content of amenorrheic and eumenorrheic athletes. N Engl J Med 1984;311:277–281.

39 Drinkwater BL, Nilson K, Ott S, Chesnut CH: Bone mineral density after resumption of menses in amenorrheic athletes. JAMA 1986;256:380–382.
40 Takada H, Washino K, Hanai T, Iwata H: Response of parathyroid hormone to exercise and bone mineral density in adolescent female athletes. Environ Health Prev Med 1998;2:161–166.
41 Tournis S, Michopoulou E, Fatouros IG, Paspati I, Michalopoulou M, Raptou P, Leontsini D, Avloniti A, Krekoukia M, Zouvelou V, Galanos A, Aggelousis N, Kambas A, Douroudos I, Lyritis GP, Taxildaris K, Pappaioannou N: Effect of rhythmic gymnastics on volumetric bone mineral density and bone geometry in premenarcheal female athletes and controls. J Clin Endocrinol Metab 2010;95:2755–2762.

Alan D. Rogol, MD, PhD
685 Explorers Road
Charlottesville, VA 22911-8441 (USA)
E-Mail adrogol@comcast.net

Lanfranco F, Strasburger CJ (eds): Sports Endocrinology.
Front Horm Res. Basel, Karger, 2016, vol 47, pp 68–81 (DOI: 10.1159/000445158)

Impact of Physical Exercise on Endocrine Aging

Joseph A.M.J.L. Janssen

Division of Endocrinology, Department of Internal Medicine, Erasmus MC, Rotterdam, The Netherlands

Abstract

Physical exercise may be vital to the maintenance of the endocrine system with aging and its helps to restore loss of activity of the endocrine system with aging. There is evidence that physical exercise induces activity of the growth hormone-insulin-like growth factor-1 axis and so produces anabolic effects in skeletal muscles. Mechano growth factor (MGF), a locally produced isoform of IGF-1, has been hypothesized to be important for the maintenance of skeletal muscles with aging. Short-term high-resistance exercise results in an increase of MGF mRNA in young but not in elderly subjects. Reported changes in levels of circulating sex steroid hormones in men after different types of (acute and chronic) physical exercise are mixed and not consistent. In addition, physical exercise may increase local effects of sex steroid hormones, and this may be more important than levels of circulating sex steroids for the maintenance and function of skeletal muscles. In elderly women, both increased physical exercise and reduced body fat may decrease levels of circulating sex hormones. Aging is further associated with changes in the dynamic functions of the hypothalamic-pituitary axis, but these changes may be attenuated/modified by aerobic training. Chronic exercise does not alter circulating cortisol levels in elderly subjects.

With aging, a progressive loss of muscle mass is found, which especially occurs in individuals with a sedentary lifestyle and low physical activity. The loss of muscle mass may result in a progressive decrease in strength and power with aging. Normally, up to the third decade, isometric and dynamic strength increase, then remains almost constant to the fifth decade of life, and then decreases with increasing age [1]. It has been found that after the age of 50 years, muscle strength drops about 30% [1]. With aging, histochemical changes occur in the muscle tissue, such as a decreased proportion and selective atrophy of type II fibers [1]. Although a decrease in muscle mass may occur in all healthy subjects with aging, acute and chronic illnesses at older age may lead to a more profound and accelerated loss of muscle mass. Reduced muscle strength may hinder the performance of common activities of daily living, and loss of muscle mass may result in dependency on others to perform one or more activities of daily living. Loss of bone mineral density and the development of osteoporosis with aging may affect both men and women. This may weaken bones so severe that accidental falls due to reduced muscle strength may lead to fractures. Aging is further characterized by reduced cardiac performance and reduced ability to perform physical activity over an extended duration of time (endurance). Aging affects nearly every hormonal gland: aging may change hormone production and secretion, e.g. decrease growth hormone (GH) secretion, which changes levels of circulating hormones, e.g. may decrease circulating insulin-like growth factor (IGF)-1; aging may further change the metabolism and degradation of hormones, e.g. less clearance/breakdown of hormones in people who have decreasing liver and/or kidney function. In addition, aging may change the sensitivity of target cells to hormones, e.g. the development of insulin resistance. The incidence of impaired glucose tolerance and type 2 diabetes are typically increasing with aging. Menopause affects women above their 40s and this induces many changes in the body, including loss of the menstrual cycle. Loss of testosterone production is associated with male aging.

With increasing age, engagement in physical activity often declines. However, regular physical exercise can minimize the physiological changes associated with aging. In addition, regular physical exercise may contribute to an improvement in overall health and well-being of an individual. Moreover, regular physical exercise may help to prevent diseases and disabilities. Benefits of regular physical activity have been proven: extensive reduction in the risk of cardiovascular disease, improvements in diabetic control, cardiac and pulmonary function as well as musculoskeletal mass, and stress reduction. In addition, regular physical exercise may be vital for the maintenance of (actions of) the endocrine system in aging. In the following section, we will first briefly discuss different types of physical training and exercise.

Types of Physical Training and Exercise

Physical exercise may improve physical performance, cardiovascular function, muscle strength, or any combination of these three [2]. There are basically two different types of physical training: aerobic training and anaerobic training, although none can be considered purely aerobic or anaerobic with respect to energy supply [2]. Aerobic training usually involves periods of continuous training (e.g. cycling or running) for a length of time at a target intensity below the anaerobic threshold [2]. In contrast, anaerobic training involves training (e.g. weight lifting, resistance training, or sprinting) at a high intensity for a short duration above the anaerobic threshold [2]. Resistance muscle strength training has often successfully been used to increase strength in elderly individuals [3]. Resistance muscle training includes exercises which combine concentric contractions (muscle shortening) and eccentric contractions (muscle lengthening) [4]. It has been reported that low-intensity resistance exercise [i.e. 40–50% of 1-RM (the repetition maximum defined as the heaviest weight you can lift if you give it your maximum effort)] is as effective as high-resistance exercise (80% of 1-RM) with regard to strength gains in individuals [5]. In the section that follows, we will discuss how physical exercise may affect (1) the GH-IGF axis, (2) sex steroids in men, (3) sex steroids in women, and (4) the hypothalamic-pituitary-adrenal axis.

Effects of Physical Exercise on the Growth Hormone-Insulin-Like Growth Factor Axis

GH and IGF-1 have important anabolic effects on protein synthesis, and thereby play a prominent role in the maintenance and improvement of muscle mass in the body [4]. In human skeletal muscle, GH and IGF-1 are involved in processes such as differentiation, hypertrophy, and angiogenesis [6]. GH is considered the major regulator of circulating IGF-1 levels, while circulating IGF-1 is predominantly synthesized by the liver [7]. After a peak in puberty, GH secretion and circulating IGF-1 levels start to decrease. Because GH is normally secreted in pulses, it is difficult to measure the 24-hour GH secretion directly. GH secretion can be measured indirectly by measuring circulating IGF-1 levels, which is considered to reflect the 24-hour secretion of GH [7]. In contrast to GH, there is little diurnal variation in circulating IGF-1 levels. Mean circulating IGF-1 levels decrease 2.5-fold by the third decade, which is followed by a further twofold decrease occurring between the third and eighth decade [7]. The age-associated decline in circulating IGF-1 levels exists even at extremely old age, without being associated with lower body mass index (BMI), hypoalbuminemia, or poor functional status.

Although the etiology of sarcopenia is multifactorial and at present not fully understood, it has been suggested that the decreases in GH secretion and circulating IGF-1 levels with aging are involved in the pathogenesis of sarcopenia [8]. Regular physical exercise may be one mechanism to increase the activity of the GH-IGF-1 axis, which may be helpful to maintain muscle mass with aging. Several studies have investigated the effects of physical exercise on GH secretion and IGF-1 levels (table 1). However, many of these studies have been performed in relatively young men. Physical exercise seems a potent stimulus for GH release. Endurance exercise elicits a greater GH response than sprint and resistance exercises. However, aging per se as well as factors associated with aging, such as the inability to achieve a sufficient absolute physical exercise intensity, results in a smaller GH response to an exercise stimulus in the elderly compared to the young [9, 10]. Based on results obtained in healthy young adults, there is evidence that circulating IGF-1 levels may increase in response to different types of physical exercise training: either aerobic, resistance exercises or heavy ergometer cycling may increase circulating IGF-1 levels [11–13]. Increased circulating IGF-1 levels after acute exercise have been found to be unrelated to exercise-

Table 1. Summary of changes in GH and IGF-1 observed during acute and chronic exercises

Reference	Study cohort	Exercise protocol	Effect
Acute studies			
Cappon et al. [38]	10 males/ 1 female	10 min above lactate threshold	Transient increase in circulating GH and IGF-1
Kraemer et al. [12]	8 males/ 8 females	Two different types of heavy-resistance exercise protocols	Circulating IGF-1 increase above rest in both males and females
Kraemer et al. [13]	6 well-trained males	Progressively intense intermittent exercise on a treadmill with finally 100% of VO_{2max}	Substantial increase in circulating GH; increase in circulating total IGF-1
Berg et al. [6]	7 females	Endurance exercise with 1 leg for 1 h	Microdialysis IGF-1 was unchanged during exercise in the exercising leg and declined after exercise
Amir et al. [23]	24 males	All-out anaerobic exercise	Transient IGF-1 elevation was significant ($p < 0.05$) only in the very fit individuals
Chronic studies			
Hambrecht et al. [16]	18 patients with chronic heart failure	6-month aerobic training intervention	Local IGF-1 expression in skeletal muscle without significant changes in systemic parameters of the GH-IGF-1 axis

induced GH secretion: for example, increasing levels of circulating IGF-1 have been reported in GH-deficient subjects. Furthermore, exercise-induced GH secretion may lead to increased local (paracrine/autocrine) IGF-1 synthesis.

Berg et al. [6] measured interstitial IGF-1 protein concentrations shortly after a single bout of aerobic physical exercise of moderate duration and observed a rapid increase in IGF-1 concentrations in skeletal muscles. Since an increase in IGF-1 protein synthesis induced by an increase in IGF-1 mRNA likely needs several hours to peak, the authors hypothesized that the observed increase in local IGF-1 levels in skeletal muscles were due to an exercise-induced mobilization of IGF-1 from local tissue stores [6]. Interestingly, they also observed higher free IGF-1 levels in the veins than in the arteries of skeletal muscles at the end of the physical exercise and shortly thereafter. They suggested this could be caused by the release of unbound IGF-1 by the skeletal muscle into the circulation [6]. However, the quantity of IGF-1 released by skeletal muscles was not sufficient to be detected in the large pool of total IGF-1 in the circulation [6]. In animal models, aerobic physical exercise has been found to be the most important intrinsic stimulus for local IGF-1 production and skeletal muscle hypertrophy [14]. In addition, in humans, it has also been found that after a single bout of mechanical loading locally produced IGF-1 mRNA increases [15]. Furthermore, it has been observed that 6 months of aerobic exercise training (also known as cardio) of patients with stable cardiac heart failure – in addition to a significant increase in oxygen uptake – may induce an increase in local (autocrine and paracrine) IGF-1 expression [16]. This increase in local (autocrine and paracrine) IGF-1 expression occurred without significant changes in the circulating parameters of the GH-IGF-1 axis [16]. Aerobic exercise training had opposite effects on the expression of local IGF-1 and the expression of the IGF-1 receptors in skeletal muscles [16]: after aerobic exercise training, local IGF-1 levels increased significantly, while IGF-1 receptor expression decreased. This latter change has been interpreted as a sign of cellular recovery of and/or reduction in local catabolic/cytotoxic factors (i.e. oxidative stress and pro-inflammatory cytokines) [16]. All these findings together suggest that aerobic exercise may augment local IGF-1 expression via GH-independent mechanisms. In corroboration of this, several studies have reported that muscle IGF-1 activity occurred without changes in circulating IGF-1 [17].

Alternative splicing of the IGF-1 gene is known to generate three different isoforms, and at least two of these have been shown to be expressed in human skeletal muscles [18]. The first isoform, IGF-1Ea, is similar in molecular structure to the (circulating) IGF-1 expressed by the liver. The second isoform, called mechano growth factor (MGF) or IGF-1Ec is expressed in response to muscle contractions and stretching [18]. It has been suggested that MGF expression in skeletal muscles peaks earlier than IGF-1 mRNA in response to muscle contractions and stretching. Muscle contractions and stretching during resistance exercises cause a preferential IGF-1 mRNA splicing towards the MGF variant. MGF is considered to be a potent local growth factor, being able to increase muscle strength by its role in activating satellite (stem cells) proliferation after muscle damage [19]. Therefore, MGF may be regarded as a repair factor.

Recently, the effects of physical exercise on the expression of IGF-1Ea and MGF in muscles were compared between young and old individuals [18]. In the resting state, no differences were observed in the expression of both isoforms between young and old individuals. However, short-term (5-week) high-resistance exercise resulted in a significant increase in MGF mRNA in the young, but not in the old individuals, while in both groups no changes in IGF-1Ea mRNA levels were observed [18]. These data suggest an attenuated MGF response to high-resistance exercise in older individuals and indicate that there is an age-related desensitization to mechanical loading [18]. However, it was also reported that after long-term (12-week) exercise of elderly people, MGF was still up-regulated [20]. Interestingly, it has also been found that administration of recombinant human GH combined with resistance exercise training can considerably increase MGF mRNA levels in the thigh muscles of elderly subjects (age 74 ± 1 years, mean ± SEM) compared to either treatment alone [20]. These data suggest that MGF mRNA levels in elderly people can be stimulated when mechanical loading in the form of resistance training is combined with administration of GH. The authors, therefore, suggested that this effect was probably reflecting a GH-mediated overall up-regulation of transcription of the IGF-1 gene prior to splicing [20].

To date, only a few studies have investigated IGF-1 responses to different forms of physical exercise in older individuals. Moreover, most studies investigating the effects of acute resistance exercises in older individuals have found no changes in circulating IGF-1. It is at present not clear whether there are stimulating effects of long-term resistance exercises on circulating IGF-1 levels in older individuals: while a number of studies have reported no changes in circulating IGF-1 levels after short-term resistance training, other studies have shown elevations of circulating IGF-1 during short-term/long-term resistance exercise programs, and this latter effect was especially observed during high-volume training. Moreover, circulating IGF-1 levels have been reported to increase in older individuals after endurance-type exercise training and after triathlon training [21]. It is unclear why circulating IGF-1 levels increase during these two forms of training. Nevertheless, it has been suggested that elevated circulating IGF-1 levels during exercise may be caused by a greater release of IGF-1 from skeletal muscles into the circulation (as a consequence of IGF-1 release from local stores by proteolytic cleavage of IGF binding proteins in skeletal muscles and greater blood flow) [22]. In anaerobic physical tests, the level of anaerobic predispositions, i.e. speed-strength abilities, is assessed by exposing subjects to a very high degree of sudden strenuous all-out exercise. Only a few data on changes in circulating IGF-1 following sudden strenuous anaerobic exercise are available in healthy older subjects. Amir et al. [23] suggested that during aging the actual fitness level is an important determinant of the effects of all-out anaerobic exercise on circulating IGF-1 levels. They demonstrated that circulating IGF-1 levels before exercise were lower in older men who were physically very fit than in older men who were physically less fit. Therefore, they suggested that muscles of physically less fit older men were more resistant to actions of IGF-1. However, when observing both fit men and less fit men, they found a transient elevation of circulating IGF-1 levels during an anaerobic physical exercise test. Nevertheless, elevations of circulating IGF-1 levels were only significant in the physically fit men. This suggests that despite the physiologically known decline in the GH-IGF-1 axis during aging, circulating IGF-1 levels may still increase in fit elderly individuals after physical exercise, while this capacity is absent (lost?) in less fit individuals. These data further suggest that during aging, the level of fitness may be an important determinant of IGF-1 responses to physical exercise. The level of fitness may thus have positive effects on aging-associated skeletal muscle loss by directly modulating the levels and actions of IGF-1.

Effects of Physical Exercise on Sex Steroids in Men

In men, sex steroid hormones are mainly secreted by the testes and the adrenals. The 'andropause' in men is characterized by a gradual decline in circulating total and bioavailable testosterone due to a decreased number of testicular Leydig cells and loss of their secretory capacity, as well as by an age-related decrease in episodic and stimulated gonadotropin secretion. In healthy men, mean circulating total testosterone

Table 2. Summary of changes in sex steroids in males during acute and chronic exercises

Reference	Study cohort	Exercise protocol	Effect
Acute studies			
Kuusi et al. [24]	20 males, healthy non-champion class joggers	Marathon (42.2 km) running	Serum levels of LH, testosterone, and SHBG all decreased
Smith et al. [39]	14 healthy active young males	Repeated sprint exercises	Increase in circulating total testosterone, free testosterone and DHT levels
Elias et al. [40]	7 physically active males	Progressive maximal-intensity physical exercise on a cycle ergometer	Transient increase in circulating testosterone
Chronic studies			
Hawkins et al. [41]	102 sedentary males	Aerobic physical exercise intervention (60 min/day for 6 days per week)	After 12 months, DHT remained +8.6% above baseline; no changes in testosterone and free testosterone

levels decrease by about 30% between age 25 and 75, whereas due to a simultaneously occurring age-associated increase in sex hormone binding globulin (SHBP) binding capacity, mean circulating free testosterone levels decrease by about 50% over this period. However, not only testosterone decreases with age, but also circulating estradiol decreases in aging males. Few observational studies have examined the association of physical exercise with sex hormones in men. Acute and chronic exercise-induced changes in circulating sex steroid hormone levels have been reported (table 2). Circulating levels of luteinizing hormone (LH), testosterone, and SHBG, all decreased during marathon running while simultaneously the serum testosterone-SHBG molar ratio, considered an index for free testosterone, did not significantly change [24]. In contrast with these findings, repeated sprint exercises (consisting of 10 repetitions of 30-second sprints at a target load of 150% of the work capacity) increased circulating total testosterone, free testosterone and dihydrotestosterone (DHT) levels in healthy active young men [25]. In another study, progressive maximal-intensity physical exercise on a cycle ergometer increased circulating testosterone levels 20 min after the beginning of the physical exercise. It was observed that circulating testosterone levels returned to baseline within 10 min of termination of physical exercise on the cycle ergometer [25]. Thus, it can be concluded that the reported changes in circulating sex steroid hormone levels during different types of physical exercise are not consistent in one direction. The different effects observed between studies on circulating sex hormone levels are probably related to differences in the study design, characteristics of the included subjects, as well as the intensity and duration of the physical exercise. In a recent study, the effect of chronic aerobic exercise on circulating sex steroid levels was tested in 102 sedentary men (aged 40–75 years). In this latter study, men were randomly assigned to an aerobic exercise intervention of moderate intensity (60 min/day, 6 days per week) or to no change in physical activity (control group). DHT increased +14.5% in the physical exercise group after 3 months compared to +1.7% in the control group ($p = 0.04$) [26]. After 12 months, DHT remained +8.6% above the baseline in the physical exercise group compared to a decrease of 3.1% in the control group ($p = 0.03$). SHBG increased 14.3% in the exercise group versus 5.7% in the control group at 3 months ($p = 0.04$), and at 12 months it remained 8.9% above the baseline in the physical exercise group versus 4.0% in the control group ($p = 0.13$). However, no statistically significant differences were observed for testosterone, free testosterone, 3α-androstanediol glucuronide, estradiol or free estradiol during 12 months between both groups [26]. Although the association between blood levels of sex hormones and prostate cancer are not well established, epidemiological studies have found that lower circulating DHT levels are associated with a decreased prostate cancer survival among men with screening-detected prostate cancer. Thus, increasing circulating DHT levels by regular physical exercise could be potentially beneficial for prostate health [26]. It has been suggested that it may be more important to focus on the tissue level of sex steroid hormones (especially in skeletal muscles) when assessing the effects of physical exercise, because both acute- and chronic-induced changes in circulating sex steroid hormone levels may not (accurately) reflect intracellular sex steroid hormone levels. In addition, recent studies have demonstrated that enzymes involved in sex hormone production (such as 17β- and 3β-hydroxysteroid dehydrogenase, 5α-reductase, and aromatase cytochrome P_{450}) are all present in skeletal muscles. As a direct consequence of the presence of these enzymes in skeletal muscles, testosterone, estradiol, and 5α-DHT may be locally synthesized from dehydroepiandrosterone and testosterone [27]. Exercise seems one way to modulate local sex steroid hormone levels in skeletal muscles. In animal and human studies, the activity of enzymes involved in sex hormone production has been found to be up-regulated in muscles by acute and chronic physical exercise [25]. Moreover, although protein expression of enzymes involved in sex hormone production was significantly lower in elderly men compared with younger men at baseline, 12 weeks of resistance exercise training significantly increased the levels of the enzymes involved in sex hormone production, and restored both serum and muscle levels of dehydroepiandrosterone, free testosterone, and DHT in older men to levels found in young subjects [28]. In this latter study, muscle steroid hormone levels were significantly correlated to muscle strength and cross-sectional area of muscles. In addition, it has been suggested that exercise-induced up-regulation of sex hormone levels in skeletal muscles during chronic physical exercise activates glucose uptake and glucose metabolism in skeletal muscles, and in this way may contribute to an improvement in glucose tolerance [29].

Table 3. Summary of changes in sex steroids during exercises in pre- and postmenopausal women

Reference	Study cohort	Exercise protocol	Effect
Premenopausal women			
Rogol et al. [42]	23 women	1-year training program at one of two exercise intensities, one at a velocity corresponding to the lactate threshold (LT) and the other halfway between that of LT and peak running velocity	A less than 2-day decrease in the luteal phase length was observed only in the greater than LT group; no significant changes for any parameter of pulsatile LH release were noted between exercise groups
Bullen et al. [43]	7 women	Moderate exercise training program (4 weeks of control, 8 weeks of training)	Reproductive hormone levels showed insignificant acute changes, and cyclic menstruation and preovulatory gonadotropin surges continued in all subjects; however, ovarian function was disturbed in 4 subjects, as evidenced by a decreased excretion of estriol, free progesterone, or both
Keizer et al. [44]	8 previously untrained eumenorrheic women	3-month endurance training program (running and cycling)	Basal luteal phase estradiol and testosterone levels were significantly lower after training; after training, testosterone increased relatively more pronounced in both the follicular and luteal phase
Bullen et al. [45]	28 previously untrained women	Subjects were expected to run 4 miles (6.4 km) per day, progressing to 10 miles (16.1 km) per day by the 5th week, and to engage daily in 3.5 h of moderate-intensity sports	32 of 53 training cycles (60%) were identifiable as abnormal by clinical assessment; loss of the positive feedback action of estrogen in 2 subjects
Postmenopausal women			
McTiernan et al. [31]	173 overweight, sedentary post-menopausal women	Moderate-intensity aerobic physical exercise program (45 min/day, 5 days/week)	Significant decrease in estradiol, estrones, and free estradiol were seen from baseline to 3 months, but this effect was attenuated after 12 months

Effects of Physical Exercise on Sex Steroids in Women

Most literature suggests that physical exercise may cause minor shifts in the hormonal milieu of premenopausal women [26] (table 3) . However, a physical exercise program of significant intensity and volume, or physical exercise combined with caloric restriction, is able to induce menstrual dysfunctions that result in decreased exposure to sex steroid hormones [26]. Observational studies have reported a delayed age at menarche, menstrual dysfunctions (amenorrhea and anovular cycles), longer menstrual cycle length, and lower progesterone and estradiol levels in athletes compared to nonathletes or sedentary women. One of the intrinsic difficulties of these observational studies is that it is almost impossible to discern individual effects of weight control and physical exercise on these results [26]. Only a few and small prospective intervention studies have been performed to investigate the effects of physical exercise on reproductive function.

The reported results are mixed: some studies reported no effects of moderate-intensity running on reproductive function while other studies reported decreased ovulation, lengthening of the menstrual cycle and menstrual dysfunctions after significant physical exercise intensity and volume [26]. Around the age of 50 years, menopause occurs in females. Cycling estradiol production from the ovarian follicles suddenly stops and very low estradiol levels remain, mainly produced by aromatization of adrenal androgens in adipose tissue. Most observational studies in postmenopausal women have found lower circulating concentrations of estradiol, estrones, and androgens during physical activity, and these effects still remained after further adjustment for BMI. It is important to note that the positive effects of physical activity on circulating sex steroid levels are closely linked to body composition as in postmenopausal women the primary source of estradiol is from aromatization of androgen precursors in adipose tissue [26]. In the Women's Health Initiative Dietary Modification Trial, women with low self-reported physical activity had higher levels of estrone, estradiol, and free estradiol than active women. The highest levels of estrogens were found in women who were both below the median level for physical activity and above the median of BMI [30]. When 173 overweight, sedentary postmenopausal women (BMI ≥24 and percent body fat >33%) were randomized to a moderate-intensity aerobic exercise program (45 min/day for 5 days per week) or to no intervention (control group), from baseline to 3 months, significant decreases in estradiol, estrone, and free estradiol levels were observed, but this effect was attenuated after 12 months (table 3). However, in women assigned to the moderate-intensity aerobic exercise program, who had still lost body fat after 12 months, the reductions in these estrogen levels still remained statistically significant [31]. Similarly, in this latter group, there was a statically significant decrease in testosterone and free testosterone compared to the control group [31]. These results suggest that in women both increased physical activity and reduced body fat may produce a decrease in circulating sex hormones. However, further studies are necessary to find out whether a physical exercise-induced decrease in circulating sex steroid levels in women has any clinical relevance (e.g. protects against sex steroid-related cancers, such as breast cancer).

Effects of Physical Exercise on the Hypothalamic-Pituitary-Adrenal Axis

Cortisol is released from the adrenal cortex in response to the stress of physical exercise. An increase in circulating cortisol levels may stimulate lipolysis in adipose cells, increase protein degradation, and decrease protein synthesis in muscle cells. This results in an increased release of glycerol, free fatty acids, and amino acids into the circulation. Cortisol is necessary for acute optimal physical exercise performance. On the other hand, physical exercise itself can be regarded as a physical stressor, and cortisol is considered a typical example of a stress-related hormone. It has been suggested that its levels increase during acute physical exercise of any intensity and decrease to normal levels in the cool-down period. The observed increase in circulating cortisol during an acute physical resistance exercise has been reported to be similar in men and women [22]. In adolescent weight lifters, the cortisol response after acute physical exercise seems to occur independent from the training status [22]. However, it has also been reported that endurance athletes show less acute cortisol response compared to acute resistance-trained men when they did the same resistance physical exercises [22]. Metabolically demanding physical exercise protocols, i.e. high-volume, moderate- to high-intensity training with short resting periods, have elicited the greatest increase in acute cortisol response, while little or no acute changes in cortisol levels were found in conventional strength/power training. Acute physical exercise programs that induce the greatest cortisol response also stimulate the greatest acute GH and lactate response. With aging, basal cortisol secretion, diurnal rhythm, and the early response to stimuli seem not to be affected, but the return to baseline values after a challenge seems delayed, probably due to diminished feedback control. This results in a prolonged exposure to cortisol and return of circulating cortisol to normal after a challenge [32]. When young (27 ± 2.8 years), older, unfit (64.6 ± 1.4 years), and older, fit (66.3 ± 2.2 years) women underwent a short bout (15 min) of treadmill exercise at high (but submaximal) intensity, the young and older women exhibited similar cortisol responses during the trial and throughout the recovery period. However, the older women had a slower decline in adrenocorticotropic hormone (ACTH) levels, suggesting that there is indeed reduced negative feedback sensitivity with aging. In addition, older, fit women had a significantly greater rate of recovery of ACTH levels compared with older, unfit women. Moreover, a significantly greater cortisol response was observed during recovery in the older, fit women compared with the older, unfit women. These results suggest that aging influences changes in the dynamic function of the hypothalamic-pituitary axis and that these latter changes may be attenuated/modified by actual physical fitness [33]. It has been hypothesized that the most plausible explanation for the greater cortisol response in the older, fit group during the recovery period is the development of a greater adrenal capacity as an adaptation to chronic physical exercise [33]. Some studies have reported that chronic exercise training does not alter circulating cortisol levels, while other studies have found significant reductions in cortisol levels during chronic exercise training. For example, when in young adults (24.8 years) with BMI ≤25 the effect of resistance physical exercises between 60 and 70% of 1-RM on circulating cortisol levels was studied, significant reductions in circulating cortisol levels were observed after 11 weeks [34]. In another study, significant reductions in circulating cortisol levels were found after 8 weeks of physical strength training in adult women (age = 22–23 years, BMI 21–22), too [35]. In contrast, no significant reductions in circulating cortisol levels have been reported in two other studies: after high-intensity physical exercises (75–85% of 1-RM) in elderly women (age = 66.1 years and BMI 26.0) [36] and after progressive strength physical training (50–80% of 1-RM) in elderly male diabetics (age = 66.6 years and BMI 28.1) [37]. The differences in mean age and BMI between study populations may (partly) explain why different effects were found in circulating cortisol levels during chronic physical exercise. On the other hand, it has been suggested that physical exercise-induced hormonal adaptations in elderly individuals need more time to show effectiveness, and it could be that the duration of the above-cited studies was too short to induce (some) hormonal adaptations [36].

Conclusions

Physical exercise may increase GH, IGF-1, and IGF-1-activated signaling pathways. There is also evidence that muscle IGF-1 may be stimulated by physical exercises. Physical exercise in the elderly may induce IGF-1 expression in the whole body and this may produce anabolic effects in skeletal muscles and thereby be an effective intervention for the prevention and treatment of sarcopenia. Simultaneously, there is also evidence that with aging there is attenuation of the ability of exercise to stimulate MGF, an isoform of IGF-1, which has been hypothesized to promote satellite (stem) cell proliferation in skeletal muscles. Interestingly, long-term exercise training in the elderly will still up-regulate MGF in skeletal muscles, and administration of GH may enhance this even further.

Acute and chronic physical exercise may induce changes in circulating sex steroid hormone levels in men. However, most studies have been performed in relatively young men and the observed effects of different types of (acute and chronic) physical exercise on sex steroid hormone levels are mixed. Differences in the study design, study population, and the intensity and duration of the physical exercise may be responsible for the reported mixed effects of physical exercise on circulating sex hormone levels. Moreover, direct effects of physical exercise on intracellular sex steroid hormone levels (especially in skeletal muscles) may play an important role in the observed positive effects of physical exercise on skeletal muscles.

Physical exercise may cause minor shifts in the hormonal milieu of premenopausal women. In postmenopausal women, both increased physical exercise and reduced body fat may produce a decrease in circulating sex hormone levels. However, it is almost impossible to disentangle the separate contribution of these two factors on circulating estradiol, since in postmenopausal women the primary source of circulating estradiol is from aromatization of androgen precursors in adipose tissue.

Cortisol is necessary for acute optimal physical exercise performance. On the other hand, physical exercise itself can be regarded as a physical stressor. Acute physical exercise may increase cortisol levels, while it has been reported that chronic physical exercise may induce no changes in circulating cortisol levels or a reduction in circulating cortisol levels. With aging, basal cortisol secretion, diurnal rhythm, and the early response to stimuli seem not to be affected, but aging is associated with changes in the dynamic function of the hypothalamic-pituitary axis, and these changes may be attenuated/modified by regular physical exercise.

References

1 Larsson L, Grimby G, Karlsson J: Muscle strength and speed of movement in relation to age and muscle morphology. J Appl Physiol Respir Environ Exerc Physiol 1979;46:451–456.

2 Radtke T, Nolan SJ, Hebestreit H, Kriemler S: Physical exercise training for cystic fibrosis. Cochrane Database Syst Rev 2015;6:CD002768.

3 Trappe S, Godard M, Gallagher P, Carroll C, Rowden G, Porter D: Resistance training improves single muscle fiber contractile function in older women. Am J Physiol Cell Physiol 2001;281:C398–C406.

4 Kraemer RR, Castracane VD: Endocrine alterations from concentric vs. eccentric muscle actions: a brief review. Metabolism 2015;64:190–201.

5 Vincent KR, Braith RW, Feldman RA, Magyari PM, Cutler RB, Persin SA, Lennon SL, Gabr AH, Lowenthal DT: Resistance exercise and physical performance in adults aged 60 to 83. J Am Geriatr Soc 2002; 50:1100–1107.

6 Berg U, Gustafsson T, Sundberg CJ, Kaijser L, Carlsson-Skwirut C, Bang P: Interstitial IGF-I in exercising skeletal muscle in women. Eur J Endocrinol 2007;157:427–435.

7 LeRoith D, Clemmons D, Nissley P, Rechler MM: NIH conference. Insulin-like growth factors in health and disease. Ann Intern Med 1992;116:854–862.

8 Butterfield GE, Thompson J, Rennie MJ, Marcus R, Hintz RL, Hoffman AR: Effect of rhGH and rhIGF-I treatment on protein utilization in elderly women. Am J Physiol 1997;272:E94–E99.

9 Gilbert KL, Stokes KA, Hall GM, Thompson D: Growth hormone responses to 3 different exercise bouts in 18- to 25- and 40- to 50-year-old men. Appl Physiol Nutr Metab 2008;33:706–712.

10 Craig BW, Brown R, Everhart J: Effects of progressive resistance training on growth hormone and testosterone levels in young and elderly subjects. Mech Ageing Dev 1989;49:159–169.

11 Cappon J, Brasel JA, Mohan S, Cooper DM: Effect of brief exercise on circulating insulin-like growth factor I. J Appl Physiol (1985) 1994;76:2490–2496.

12 Kraemer WJ, Gordon SE, Fleck SJ, Marchitelli LJ, Mello R, Dziados JE, Friedl K, Harman E, Maresh C, Fry AC: Endogenous anabolic hormonal and growth factor responses to heavy resistance exercise in males and females. Int J Sports Med 1991;12:228–235.

13 Kraemer RR, Durand RJ, Acevedo EO, Johnson LG, Kraemer GR, Hebert EP, Castracane VD: Rigorous running increases growth hormone and insulin-like growth factor-I without altering ghrelin. Exp Biol Med (Maywood) 2004;229:240–246.

14 McKoy G, Ashley W, Mander J, Yang SY, Williams N, Russell B, Goldspink G: Expression of insulin growth factor-1 splice variants and structural genes in rabbit skeletal muscle induced by stretch and stimulation. J Physiol 1999;516:583–592.

15 Bamman MM, Shipp JR, Jiang J, Gower BA, Hunter GR, Goodman A, McLafferty CL Jr, Urban RJ: Mechanical load increases muscle IGF-I and androgen receptor mRNA concentrations in humans. Am J Physiol Endocrinol Metab 2001;280:E383–E390.

16 Hambrecht R, Schulze PC, Gielen S, Linke A, Mobius-Winkler S, Erbs S, Kratzsch J, Schubert A, Adams V, Schuler G: Effects of exercise training on insulin-like growth factor-I expression in the skeletal muscle of non-cachectic patients with chronic heart failure. Eur J Cardiovasc Prev Rehabil 2005;12:401–406.

17 Adams GR: Role of insulin-like growth factor-I in the regulation of skeletal muscle adaptation to increased loading. Exerc Sport Sci Rev 1998;26:31–60.

18 Hameed M, Orrell RW, Cobbold M, Goldspink G, Harridge SD: Expression of IGF-I splice variants in young and old human skeletal muscle after high resistance exercise. J Physiol 2003;547:247–254.

19 Hill M, Wernig A, Goldspink G: Muscle satellite (stem) cell activation during local tissue injury and repair. J Anat 2003;203:89–99.

20 Hameed M, Lange KH, Andersen JL, Schjerling P, Kjaer M, Harridge SD, Goldspink G: The effect of recombinant human growth hormone and resistance training on IGF-I mRNA expression in the muscles of elderly men. J Physiol 2004;555:231–240.

21 Moran S, Chen YM, Ruthie A, Nir Y: Alterations in IGF-I affect elderly: role of physical activity. Eur Rev Aging Phys Act 2007;4:77–84.

22 Kraemer WJ, Ratamess NA: Hormonal responses and adaptations to resistance exercise and training. Sports Med 2005;35:339–361.

23 Amir R, Ben-Sira D, Sagiv M: IGF-I and FGF-2 responses to Wingate anaerobic test in older men. J Sports Sci Med 2007;6:227–232.

24 Kuusi T, Kostiainen E, Vartiainen E, Pitkanen L, Ehnholm C, Korhonen HJ, Nissinen A, Puska P: Acute effects of marathon running on levels of serum lipoproteins and androgenic hormones in healthy males. Metabolism 1984;33:527–531.

25 Sato K, Iemitsu M: Exercise and sex steroid hormones in skeletal muscle. J Steroid Biochem Mol Biol 2015;145:200–205.

26 McTiernan A: Mechanisms linking physical activity with cancer. Nat Rev Cancer 2008;8:205–211.

27 Aizawa K, Iemitsu M, Maeda S, Jesmin S, Otsuki T, Mowa CN, Miyauchi T, Mesaki N: Expression of steroidogenic enzymes and synthesis of sex steroid hormones from DHEA in skeletal muscle of rats. Am J Physiol Endocrinol Metab 2007;292:E577–E584.

28 Sato K, Iemitsu M, Matsutani K, Kurihara T, Hamaoka T, Fujita S: Resistance training restores muscle sex steroid hormone steroidogenesis in older men. FASEB J 2014;28:1891–1897.
29 Sato K, Iemitsu M, Aizawa K, Mesaki N, Fujita S: Increased muscular dehydroepiandrosterone levels are associated with improved hyperglycemia in obese rats. Am J Physiol Endocrinol Metab 2011;301:E274–E280.
30 McTiernan A, Wu L, Chen C, Chlebowski R, Mossavar-Rahmani Y, Modugno F, Perri MG, Stanczyk FZ, Van Horn L, Wang CY; Women's Health Initiative Investigators: Relation of BMI and physical activity to sex hormones in postmenopausal women. Obesity (Silver Spring) 2006;14:1662–1677.
31 McTiernan A, Tworoger SS, Rajan KB, Yasui Y, Sorenson B, Ulrich CM, Chubak J, Stanczyk FZ, Bowen D, Irwin ML, Rudolph RE, Potter JD, Schwartz RS: Effect of exercise on serum androgens in postmenopausal women: a 12-month randomized clinical trial. Cancer Epidemiol Biomarkers Prev 2004;13:1099–1105.
32 Sapolsky RM, Krey LC, McEwen BS: The neuroendocrinology of stress and aging: the glucocorticoid cascade hypothesis. Endocr Rev 1986;7:284–301.
33 Traustadottir T, Bosch PR, Cantu T, Matt KS: Hypothalamic-pituitary-adrenal axis response and recovery from high-intensity exercise in women: effects of aging and fitness. J Clin Endocrinol Metab 2004;89:3248–3254.
34 Izquierdo M, Ibanez J, Gonzalez-Badillo JJ, Hakkinen K, Ratamess NA, Kraemer WJ, French DN, Eslava J, Altadill A, Asiain X, Gorostiaga EM: Differential effects of strength training leading to failure versus not to failure on hormonal responses, strength, and muscle power gains. J Appl Physiol (1985) 2006;100:1647–1656.
35 Marx JO, Ratamess NA, Nindl BC, Gotshalk LA, Volek JS, Dohi K, Bush JA, Gomez AL, Mazzetti SA, Fleck SJ, Hakkinen K, Newton RU, Kraemer WJ: Low-volume circuit versus high-volume periodized resistance training in women. Med Sci Sports Exerc 2001;33:635–643.
36 Vale RG, de Oliveira RD, Pernambuco CS, de Meneses YP, Novaes Jda S, de Andrade Ade F: Effects of muscle strength and aerobic training on basal serum levels of IGF-1 and cortisol in elderly women. Arch Gerontol Geriatr 2009;49:343–347.
37 Ibanez J, Gorostiaga EM, Alonso AM, Forga L, Arguelles I, Larrion JL, Izquierdo M: Lower muscle strength gains in older men with type 2 diabetes after resistance training. J Diabetes Complications 2008;22:112–118.
38 Cappon J, Brasel JA, Mohan S, Cooper DM: Effect of brief exercise on circulating insulin-like growth factor I. J Appl Physiol (1985) 1994;76:2490–2496.
39 Smith AA, Toone R, Peacock O, Drawer S, Stokes KA, Cook CJ: Dihydrotestosterone is elevated following sprint exercise in healthy young men. J Appl Physiol (1985) 2013;114:1435–1440.
40 Elias AN, Wilson AF, Pandian MR, Rojas FJ, Kayaleh R, Stone SC, James N: Melatonin and gonadotropin secretion after acute exercise in physically active males. Eur J Appl Physiol Occup Physiol 1993;66:357–361.
41 Hawkins VN, Foster-Schubert K, Chubak J, Sorensen B, Ulrich CM, Stancyzk FZ, Plymate S, Stanford J, White E, Potter JD, McTiernan A: Effect of exercise on serum sex hormones in men: a 12-month randomized clinical trial. Med Sci Sports Exerc 2008;40:223–233.
42 Rogol AD, Weltman A, Weltman JY, Seip RL, Snead DB, Levine S, Haskvitz EM, Thompson DL, Schurrer R, Dowling E, et al: Durability of the reproductive axis in eumenorrheic women during 1 yr of endurance training. J Appl Physiol (1985) 1992;72:1571–1580.
43 Bullen BA, Skrinar GS, Beitins IZ, Carr DB, Reppert SM, Dotson CO, Fencl MD, Gervino EV, McArthur JW: Endurance training effects on plasma hormonal responsiveness and sex hormone excretion. J Appl Physiol Respir Environ Exerc Physiol 1984;56:1453–1463.
44 Keizer HA, Kuipers H, de Haan J, Janssen GM, Beckers E, Habets L, van Kranenburg G, Geurten P: Effect of a 3-month endurance training program on metabolic and multiple hormonal responses to exercise. Int J Sports Med 1987;8(suppl 3):154–160.
45 Bullen BA, Skrinar GS, Beitins IZ, von Mering G, Turnbull BA, McArthur JW: Induction of menstrual disorders by strenuous exercise in untrained women. N Engl J Med 1985;312:1349–1353.

Joseph A.M.J.L. Janssen, MD, PhD
Department of Internal Medicine, Erasmus MC
Room D-443, 's-Gravendijkwal 230
NL–3015 CE Rotterdam (The Netherlands)
E-Mail j.a.m.j.l.janssen@erasmusmc.nl

Use of Performance-Enhancing Endocrine Drugs (Doping) in Competitive and Recreational Sports Activity

Lanfranco F, Strasburger CJ (eds): Sports Endocrinology.
Front Horm Res. Basel, Karger, 2016, vol 47, pp 82–100 (DOI: 10.1159/000445159)

Androgens

Rakesh Iyer • David J. Handelsman

Department of Andrology, Concord Repatriation General Hospital, and ANZAC Research Institute, University of Sydney, Sydney, N.S.W., Australia

Abstract

Androgen abuse is the most potent and prevalent form of sports doping detected. It originated from the early years of the Cold War as an epidemic confined to drug cheating within elite power sports. In the decades following the end of the Cold War, it has become disseminated into an endemic based within the illicit drug subcultures serving recreational abusers seeking cosmetic body sculpting effects. Within sports, both direct androgen abuse (administration of androgens), as well as indirect androgen abuse (administration of nonandrogenic drugs to increase endogenous testosterone), is mostly readily detectable with mass spectrometry-based anti-doping urine tests. The ongoing temptation of fame and fortune and the effectiveness of androgen abuse in power sports continue to entice cheating via renewed approaches aiming to exploit androgens. These require ongoing vigilance, inventiveness in anti-doping science, and targeting coaches as well as athletes in order to build resilience against doping and maintain fairness in elite sport. The challenge of androgen abuse in the community among recreational abusers has barely been recognized and effective approaches remain to be developed.

Androgens are a class of hormones based on the two canonical endogenous steroids, testosterone (T) and its potent metabolite, dihydrotestosterone (DHT). Androgen effects are produced by binding to, and activating, the androgen receptor (AR) resulting in the development and maintenance of the male reproductive system as well as characteristic nonreproductive effects on classical androgen target tissues such as muscle, skin, and bone, and more subtle effects on most other somatic tissues which ubiquitously express AR [1]. Androgen binding to AR protein results in conformational AR changes, liberation from chaperone protein binding, and AR dimerization which facilitates binding to androgen-response elements in target genes. This allows attachment of coregulators to regulate characteristic patterns of gene expression that represent the actions of androgens [2]. In addition, nongenomic effects of androgens, mediated by postulated non-AR, membrane-binding mechanisms, are widely discussed but not yet well characterized [3].

Testosterone

T was first fully characterized as the principal male sex steroid of testicular origin in 1935 [4] followed rapidly by its first clinical use (1937) [5] and a Nobel Prize (1939). Following the hiatus of World War II, the pharmaceutical industry development of synthetic steroids included pursuing the goal of a nonvirilizing androgen ('anabolic steroid') potentially suitable for use to obtain pharmacological androgen effects in women and children. Contrasting with the successful development of synthetic glucocorticoids and oral contraceptives during the golden age of steroid pharmacology, the industrial quest for an 'anabolic steroid' based on dissociating the virilizing from the anabolic effects of androgens failed. This is now understood in the light of the later discovery of the singular AR together with the flawed interpretations of relatively nonspecific whole animal bioassays then used to screen synthetic steroids for supposedly distinct anabolic and virilizing effects. Yet, despite the industry's abandonment of this fruitless endeavor by 1980, and its recent reincarnation under the guise of developing a 'selective AR modulator' (SARM) [6], the empty concept of an 'anabolic steroid' persists as an ill-defined and misleading scientific terminology [7, 8]. In this paper, the more accurate and clearer term 'androgen' is used exclusively for both endogenous and synthetic androgens, but includes references to chemicals loosely defined elsewhere as 'anabolic steroids' or 'anabolic-androgenic steroids', which confuse by making an obsolete distinction where there is no difference.

The primary therapeutic indication for T is in replacement therapy for men with disorders of the reproductive system that prevent normal synthesis of T. This may be due to either testicular damage that disrupts Leydig cell T synthesis and secretion, or hypothalamo-pituitary disorders which limit pituitary LH secretion that drives Leydig cell T production. The major limitation of T as a therapeutic drug is its short duration of action and minimal oral bioactivity due to first-pass hepatic metabolism. For T replacement therapy, these limitations were overcome by creation of long-acting depot injectable T formed by T esterified with lipophilic, long-chain fatty acids formulated in a vegetable oil vehicle [9]. These remained the most widely used T products for decades until the more recent advent of transdermal gels delivering unesterified T.

Synthetic Androgens

During the postwar decades, thousands of synthetic androgens were invented based on the steroidal structures of the natural androgens, T, and DHT [10]. The vast majority were subjected to 17-α alkylation, which rendered androgens more potent and orally active but suffered from class-specific hepatotoxicity, an adverse effect not shared by endogenous androgens or other classes of synthetic androgens. Only a tiny minority of these synthetic androgens outlined in the pharmaceutical patent literature of the 1950s–1970s were ever marketed. Many more, never-marketed androgens were described and evaluated in research laboratories with no or only preliminary clinical studies.

Due to their hepatotoxicity, most marketed synthetic 17-α alkylated androgens have been progressively eliminated from the market [11]. Yet the ergogenic advantages of androgens for power sports and their efficacy for body sculpting fostered the continuing availability of well-known alkylated androgens such as stanozolol, methandienone and oxandrolone via the internet for illicit use [12–17]. However, in sports, all marketed androgens were readily identified by mass spectrometry (MS)-based doping detection methods [10] making such androgen doping highly risky. Consequently, various alternative strategies were adopted to continue exploiting androgen doping without detection by other means. One approach has been to utilize never-marketed synthetic androgens identified from the old patent literature, but whose structures were unfamiliar and undisclosed while MS-based urine detection tests required a known structure [15, 18, 19]. The first such designer androgen identified in an athlete's urine was norbolethone, a 17-α alkylated androgen originally synthesized in 1960 but never marketed [20]. Soon after, tetrahydrogestrinone, a previously unknown androgen produced illicitly by a one-step chemical reduction of a marketed alkylated progestin (gestrinone) was identified structurally [21] and then as a potent androgen by an in vitro androgen bioassay [22]. Subsequently, desoxymethyltestosterone (Madol), another never-marketed androgen patented in the 1960s, was identified [23]. A recent review notes at least six designer androgens available over the internet [17]. Nevertheless, once identified, these designer androgens have never again been detected in regular doping tests reflecting effective deterrence. More broadly, similar never-marketed androgens are also commonly found in unregulated, over-the-counter and internet-marketed food supplements, which often do not identify steroids on the label but are promoted as purportedly legal body-building alternatives to androgens [15, 24].

The first nonsteroidal androgen invented was reported in 1998 [25] leading to a new class of structurally diverse AR agonists (SARM) with the overall goal of tissue selectivity, reviving the older attempts to dissociate virilizing from anabolic effects of androgens [6]. This aims to replicate the serendipitous but largely unexplained tissue selectivity of selective estrogen receptor modulators (SERMs). So far, nonsteroidal androgens are not yet approved for clinical use [26–28] and their use in sport was prohibited in 2008. Yet, characteristically, potentially ergogenic drugs in premarketing development become available illicitly over the internet for doping or body building, in breach of law, patents, and doping codes. For example, Andarine (S-4), widely advertised on the internet [29], has been identified in urine samples from athletes [30, 31]. Given the limited clinical trial data available [27], the full safety profile of nonsteroidal androgens, even at conventional let alone doping doses, remains little understood.

Efficacy of Androgen Abuse

The ergogenic effects of androgen doping in eugonadal men were long doubted with the claimed benefits attributed to placebo effects of expectation, athletic training, and nutrition. Even meta-analyses of controlled studies were misleadingly negative [32] as they were restricted, by perceived ethical constraints, to conventional androgen doses but failed to reproduce the supraphysiological doses used in doping. In 1996, Bhasin et al. [33] unequivocally proved that administration of T at supraphysiological doses increased fat-free mass, muscle size, and strength in eugonadal normal men without, but also in addition to, exercise. Unequivocally, this improves performance in power sports although the influence on endurance or skill-dependent sports is less clear [34]. In addition to the myotrophic effects, the main goal of androgen doping, supraphysiological doses of T or synthetic androgens also elevate hemoglobin levels [35], mood, motivation, and aggression [36], and exert neural effects on the regulation of muscle functions [37–39], all of which may augment the ergogenic effects.

History of Androgen Abuse: From Epidemic to Endemic

Androgen abuse in sports originated during the early years of the Cold War among elite athletes of Eastern European countries as a short-cut scheme to demonstrate symbolic supremacy over their Western political rivals [7, 18]. This led to systematic national doping programs with the East German program disclosed after the fall of the Berlin Wall [40] although comparable national programs of other Eastern bloc countries remain undisclosed. Ultimately, androgen doping was enthusiastically but surreptitiously adopted by elite athletes and coaches from competing nations reaching epidemic proportions in certain sports, notably power sports where the gains in muscle mass and strength were most advantageous and especially conspicuous among female athletes [40].

Towards the end of the Cold War among countries with sustainable illicit drug subculture networks, androgen abuse spread from elite power sports to the larger market of recreational users for cosmetic effects. By the 1990s, this had transformed an epidemic focused on elite power sports into a new, endemic dimension of illicit urban drug consumption easily grafted onto body beautiful and image enhancement subcultures. During the preceding decade, this progression was propelled by

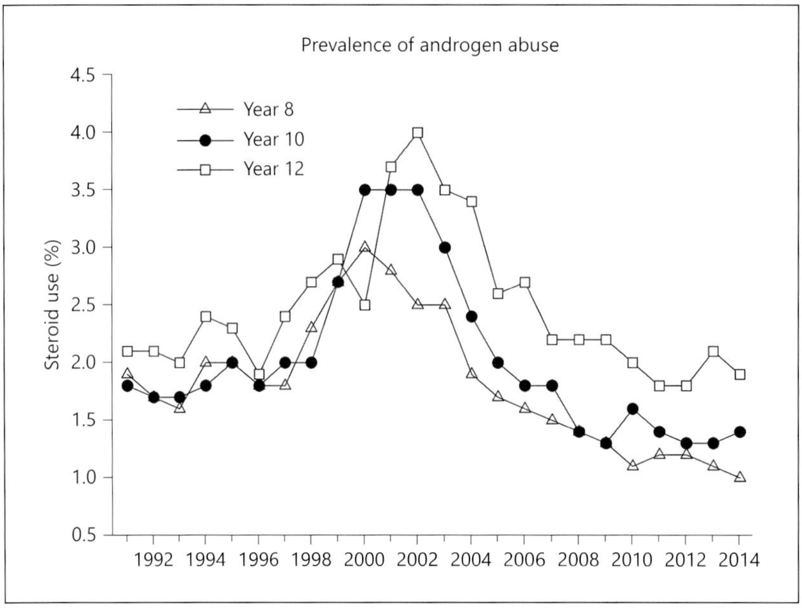

Fig. 1. Prevalence of 'steroid' use (ever) admitted in serial standardized anonymous questionnaire surveys among secondary school students in years 8, 10 and 12 of a stratified random sample of US high schools (adapted from Monitoring the Future surveys [52]).

entrepreneurial drug dealers fostering an underground folklore, epitomized by the infamous *Underground Steroid Handbook* of the early 1980s and culminating in the present situation where the majority of current androgen abusers now aim to achieve cosmetic goals such as body building and/or image sculpting for recreational or occupational reasons rather than sports doping [41, 42]. An important prospective stratified random sampling study provides evidence that, among US adolescents, the prevalence of androgen abuse may have peaked at the turn of the 21st century and been declining since (fig. 1).

Therapeutic Use Exemption

The International Olympic Committee (IOC) recognized the issues of doping by releasing the first list of prohibited drugs in 1967 and instituting detection testing in 1974. Subsequently, it fostered the establishment in 1999 of the World Anti-Doping Agency (WADA) to carry the responsibility for anti-doping prohibition, deterrence, and detection through enacting the WADA Code, a harmonized set of global rules to prohibit and prevent doping in sports [43]. The WADA Code mandates a strict liability in prohibiting drug use (including attempted use, possession, trade, and sample tampering or test avoidance) rendering the presence of a banned drug in the body as an anti-doping rule violation, regardless of intent, fault, negligence, or knowing use.

One consequence of this strict liability is that it is necessary to make provision for the rare athlete who suffers from T deficiency due to genuine pathological disorders of the reproductive system [44]. Applications for therapeutic use exemption are reviewed by independent medical experts based on detailed medical reports documenting the athlete's disorder. The criteria that must be satisfied include proving the need for the banned drug, that there is no nonbanned alternative, and that the treatment, notably dosage, would provide no ergogenic advantage. Therapeutic use exemptions for T must be approved prior to administration with the approval based on a well-documented medical history of conditions such as pituitary tumors and their treatment, or testicular pathology such as bilateral orchidectomy, genetic disorders (anorchia or Klinefelter's syndrome), infections (orchitis) or toxin-induced effects (chemotherapy, radiotherapy, or other cytotoxic testicular damage) [45]. By contrast, functional states with a low serum T level due to prior androgen abuse, overtraining, aging or nonreproductive disorders are not acceptable.

Prevalence of Androgen Abuse

Androgens are the most potent and most frequently detected doping agents in elite sports. Owing to their prominent effects on muscle mass and strength, androgens are particularly effective in power sports such as weight lifting, combat sports, sprinting, and throwing [34]. The majority of positive doping tests recorded in WADA's 32 approved national anti-doping laboratories are attributable to androgens. In 2013, among the total of 269,878 samples analyzed, 2.2% had either adverse analytical findings (1.3%) – which are presumptive anti-doping rule violations – or atypical findings (0.9%), with nearly two thirds of positive tests due to androgen doping, six times higher than the next category of prohibited drugs [46]. While data on current doping would not be a proper estimate of the overall prevalence of elite athletes who have ever doped, they do imply the testing regimen provides effective deterrence of androgen doping, at least during elite sports competition, which accounts for most tests. As expected, more sophisticated sampling strategies for deviant or illicit behaviors suggest a higher prevalence of ever-use of doping drugs compared with lower rates of current use in objective testing [47, 48] although anonymized estimates that do not itemize the doping methods may inflate estimates if athletes mistakenly include nonbanned supplements as 'doping' [49]. In theory, greater coverage by out-of-competition testing and/or refined detection of long-term androgen metabolites to widen the time window of detection can further enhance the detection of androgen doping during training periods before competition. The predominance of androgens among positive doping tests also reflects the difficulties in detecting doping with either proteins such as erythropoietin, growth hormone, or growth hormone-releasing peptides, or autologous blood doping, which are believed to be more widely used in endurance and contact sports than has been routinely detected so far. Detection of peptide hormone doping is hampered by relatively short time windows of detection resulting in likely underestimation of the true current or ever prevalence of peptide and hemoglobin doping to a much greater extent than for androgen doping.

In recent decades, androgen abuse has become an established endemic in affluent countries. A recent meta-analysis of 187 studies estimated the global lifetime prevalence of androgen abuse in the general population as 3.3% with the prevalence 4 times higher in men (6.4%) than women (1.6%) [50]. Androgen abuse is more prevalent among athletes compared with nonathletes and in recreational compared with elite competitors. However, prevalence estimates from questionnaire-based surveys may be inflated by ambiguity in self-reports of 'steroid' use confusing it with nonandrogens (e.g. glucocorticoids for asthma) or over-the-counter food supplements [49]. In the wider community, based on stratified random sampling methodology, androgen abuse among non-elite athletes is claimed to begin in high school years [51, 52], but later than for most other illicit drugs [53], and to mostly subside by the 3rd decade of life [52], leaving a small subgroup of older androgen abusers with prominent psychological disorders including alcohol and other drug abuse [54]. Recent US surveys suggest that adolescent androgen abuse may have peaked around the turn of the 21st century with decreasing prevalence over the past 15 years [7, 52]. The prevalence of community-based androgen abuse also appears to vary markedly according to geographical location, with highest prevalence reported in the Middle East and South America, as well as among immigrants within a country [55], findings suggesting the influence of psychosocial and economic factors [50].

Types of Androgen Doping: Direct and Indirect

Androgen doping may be either direct or indirect. Direct androgen doping involves administration of endogenous or synthetic androgens. It initially involved use of marketed synthetic androgens including exogenous natural androgens such as T and DHT, but more recently has extended to nonmarketed synthetic designer and nutraceutical androgens. Direct androgen doping using synthetic androgens is now readily detected in urine samples using gas or liquid chromatography, MS-based methods subject only to knowing the chemical structure of the administered drug and ideally its metabolite profiles. In many instances, the window of detection is already sensitive and wide, up to months since the last dose, leading to the reverse problem – that of athletes claiming an inadvertent source of the prohibited steroids from dietary consumption of contaminated meat or other food products [56–58].

Indirect doping refers to administration of nonandrogenic drugs that increase endogenous T with a view to gaining ergogenic advantage or to reverse the deleterious effects of reproductive axis suppression resulting from androgen doping [59]. The drugs used for indirect androgen doping include hCG and LH, anti-estrogens including estrogen receptor antagonists or estrogen synthesis (aromatase) inhibitors. In addition to nonsteroidal drugs, a limited number of steroids consisting of natural androgen precursors (or pro-androgens) like dehydroepiandrosterone (DHEA) or androstenedione (A) that are converted to T and/or DHT in the body, or epitestosterone (E) used to mask the T/E ratio, may also be considered as indirect androgen doping [60].

Both hCG and LH are members of the pituitary glycoprotein hormone family with TSH and FSH, all being heterodimers that share a common α-subunit with distinctive β-subunits that confer the target receptor specificity and bioactivity. LH and hCG have highly homologous β-subunits and act on the same common CG/LH receptor, expressed primarily on testicular Leydig cells and ovarian follicle theca cells. Physiologically, hCG is secreted only by the placenta and is normally undetectable in the serum or urine of men, rendering positive results an abnormal finding. hCG features a C-terminal extension of 22 amino acids including 4 O-linked carbohydrate side chains that extend its circulating half-life compared with LH which has a very brief circulating half-life. Hence, therapeutically, hCG is a convenient, natural long-acting analogue of LH given at daily or longer intervals whereas LH would require multiple daily injections. Therapeutic-grade hCG is either purified from human pregnancy urine or produced in vitro by genetic engineering of mammalian cells in culture as a recombinant glycoprotein. Pituitary LH, once extracted from human cadaveric pituitaries, is no longer available since 1985 when deaths from Creutzfeldt-Jakob disease were reported due to administration of contaminated pituitary gonadotropins [61]; more recently, recombinant LH is marketed when produced by the same methods as recombinant hCG. The sole therapeutic indication for hCG in men is to restore normal serum T concentration and androgen status in gonadotropin-deficient men undergoing induction of spermatogenesis and fertility [59, 62]. By contrast, LH has no therapeutic indication in men whereas in women both hCG and LH are used as ovulation triggers during infertility treatments.

In men, hCG administration produces a sustained increase in endogenous T production with increased serum and urine T concentrations [63]. This leads to suppression of serum and urine LH, which may be useful corroborative findings to confirm suspected exogenous hCG use, whereas the urine T/E ratio, a marker for exogenous T use, is unaffected by hCG use [63, 64]. By contrast, recombinant LH appears to be an ineffective doping agent as administration is unable to increase serum or urine T even at very high (32 times recommended) dose [63]. This lack of efficacy coupled with the need for multiple daily injections and high cost render it implausible as a genuine doping threat although vigilance is still required to detect and deter even irrational doping efforts.

Effective estrogen blockade has potential ergogenic effects through creating a reflex rise in endogenous T production. This arises by blocking part of the T-induced negative feedback inhibition of the hypothalamus-pituitary regulation of pituitary LH secretion which relies on aromatization of T to estradiol. The relevant drugs include the older estrogen receptor antagonists, clomiphene and tamoxifen, together with many newer estrogen receptor blocking congeners, the so-called SERMs, estrogen receptor mixed agonists/antagonists with distinctively different tissue impact that depend on still not understood mechanisms dictating different tissue specificity [65]. More recently, estrogen synthesis (aromatase) inhibitors, developed primarily for breast cancer therapeutics, block enzymatic synthesis of estradiol from T by the enzyme aromatase [66]. While rarely used off-label for the treatment of gynecomastia, estrogen blockers are promoted in the doping folklore to reverse the suppressive effects of long-term androgen abuse in suppressing the hypothalamo-pituitary testicular axis. However, increases in serum LH and T may not be sustained even during prolonged estrogen blockade and, in any case, this maintains and prolongs the underlying gonadal axis suppression while merely deferring and possibly retarding recovery [67]. By contrast, estrogen blockade has negligible effect on blood T concentrations in women [59].

Patterns and Motivation of Androgen Abuse

Patterns of androgen abuse vary according to the goal (type of sports or body building) and local drug folklore and availability. Common patterns include cycling, stacking, or pyramiding in the belief that these patterns maximize ergogenic advantage while reducing side effects and, for doping, risk of detection. The common feature is the ingestion of multiple drugs with purportedly different and synergistic properties to amplify gains in muscle mass and strength [41, 42, 68] but ultimately involving massive (up to 29 times recommended) doses [68]. History shows that, in order to properly appraise the medical risks and benefits of androgen abuse, it is essential, even if challenging, to replicate the actual androgen abuse patterns.

Cycling is characterized by 'on' and 'off' periods of steroid use [69], a practice used more by athletes seeking competitive ergogenic advantage, whereas noncompetitive body builders, lacking concern for detection, more often use androgen continuously. The rationale for intermittent rather than continuous treatment, interspersed with periods of nonuse, is apparently to allow for recovery of sensitivity following the desensitization due to the high-dose androgen exposure. While there is no direct, objective evidence of such desensitization, it is plausible and preliminary attempts to incorporate intermittent T treatment into therapeutics are reported [70, 71].

Androgen abusers often combine other drugs for synergism and/or to reverse side effects. Growth hormone, its secretagogues, and erythropoietin may be combined for synergistic ergogenic effects, depending on the sport. hCG or estrogen blockade is used to counter the suppression of the hypothalamo-pituitary-testicular axis which causes reduction in testicular size, spermatogenesis and male infertility, although these regimens would also delay recovery from the underlying hypothalamic suppression. Estrogen blockade is also sought to treat androgen-induced gynecomastia while androgen-induced acne may be treated with broad-spectrum antibiotics, 5α-reductase inhibitors or retinoids, and the 5α-reductase inhibitors may also be sought for male-pattern balding.

An important dimension of deterring doping is a better understanding of the social and psychological motivations of the doping athlete. Well-designed psychological primary prevention programs aiming to deter adolescent athletes from future doping behavior have proven effective at increasing knowledge but not reducing doping intentions or behavior [72]. This approach may have failed due to overlooking the role of coaches as privileged advisors, who exert decisive influence on athletes including their susceptibility to and practice of doping. In a highly competitive environment laced with high temptations of fame and fortune status, a key driver of doping, which athletes understand is dishonest and unhealthy and risks banning, is the so-called 'false consensus effect' whereby the belief that their competitors are cheating, based on usually unfounded, self-justifying suspicions and rumors, rationalizes cheating [73]. A heightened awareness of the coaches' role in doping susceptibility and practice is targeted in the widening responsibilities of the athlete's entourage under the new 2015 WADA Code, and research programs aimed at coaches as decisive facilitators of promoting (or undermining) fairness are warranted.

Laboratory Detection of Androgen Abuse

The IOC's prohibition of androgens in the 1970s made the development of corresponding testing necessary to enforce the prohibition by detecting and deterring use of banned steroids. At that time, while the steroid immunoassay was becoming the dominant clinical technology for its speed, throughput, and affordability, its major drawback of suboptimal specificity, which depended on the antibody for the degree of cross-reaction with the numerous possible structurally related steroids, rendered it inadequate for anti-doping tests, where a positive test had dire consequences for a professional athlete. Laboratory detection of androgen abuse has developed highly sensitive and specific gas or liquid chromatography, MS urine tests by which means any synthetic androgen will be detectable once its chemical structure is known. Among the adverse analytical findings reported in 2013 from WADA's anti-doping laboratories, 36 different synthetic androgens were detected [46]. Ongoing research is identifying longer-term metabolites of synthetic androgens to further widen the window of detection [74–76]. The high risk of detection, as shown by the low incidence of positives for synthetic androgens, provides a strong deterrent to their use for all but ill-advised athletes. Nevertheless, androgens remain such potent ergogenic drugs that elite athletes and their coaches willing to cheat if they can escape detection have adopted various devious approaches to continue exploiting this unfair advantage. These include using previously unknown synthetic androgens whose undisclosed chemical structures make MS detection difficult as well as use of exogenous administration of natural androgens or their precursors (pro-androgens) which are difficult to distinguish from their endogenous counterparts. The unrecognized synthetic androgens include the so-called designer or nutraceutical androgens selected to be difficult to detect and/or included in unregulated food supplements without label disclosure. However, once identified, these steroids are readily added to the Prohibited List together with suitable detection tests and, of the various designer androgens identified, none has ever been detected again. Nevertheless, the profusion of different synthetic androgens harbored in the patent literature of the 1960s and 1970s creates a formidable ongoing, although theoretically tractable, task.

Given the effective deterrence for use of known synthetic androgens, the majority (60%) of adverse analytical findings for androgens are now for use of natural androgens, notably T [46]. Use of exogenous natural androgens and pro-androgens such as T, DHT, A, DHEA, and E for doping creates important additional difficulty to distinguish between endogenous and exogenous versions of the same molecule which cannot be distinguished from their endogenous counterparts by conventional MS. The first approach to detecting exogenous use of T has been to measure the urine T/E ratio, which depends on the coproduction of both T and its biologically inactive, 17α-epimer E by Leydig cells. In theory, administration of exogenous T sufficient to reduce Leydig cell production of both T and E would increase the urine T/E ratio, providing a marker for exogenous T use. While E production rate is <5% of T, its rapid excretion in urine makes the urine T/E ratio, determined from the excreted glucuronidated metabolites, results in a relatively stable within-individual T/E ratio with a Caucasian population mean of ~1 and a 99% upper confidence limit of ~4 [60].

One limitation of the urine T/E ratio is the common genetic deletion polymorphism of the phase II hepatic enzyme, uridine diphosphate glucuronyl transferase (UGT)2B17, which renders T more hydrophilic by glucuronidation to facilitate urinary excretion [77]. The homozygous deletion of UGT2B17 results in a major reduction in T glucuronidation so that those individuals have a population mean urine T/E ratio of ~0.1, creating a false negative which could mask exogenous T administration [78]. This challenge is met by the introduction of the Athlete's Biological Passport [79] implementing a Bayesian model of serial adaptive individual-based reference limits to supplant population-based reference limits [80]. Whether additional knowledge of the UGT2B17 genotype is useful beyond the T/E ratio phenotype remains to be defined [78]. An alternative or corroborative marker for the administration of any exogenous androgen is the urine T/LH ratio [63, 64, 81]; however, this measure depends on the validity of urine LH measurements by immunoassays which are validated solely for human serum samples so that they suffer from method-specific bias and only a few are valid for human urine measurements [82].

An important tool for detecting administration of exogenous natural androgens is the carbon isotope MS which measures the $^{13}C/^{12}C$ ratio of urinary excreted T. This depends on the observation that commercial production of steroids uses, as a starting material, plant sterols that have a lower (depleted) $^{13}C/^{12}C$ ratio due to differences between photosynthetic and mammalian steroid synthesis pathways. Hence, the administration of a commercially sourced exogenous T product accordingly lowers the $^{13}C/^{12}C$ ratio in urinary T compared with excreted endogenous T. A significantly low

$^{13}C/^{12}C$ ratio in urinary T is indicative of exogenous T administration. An analogous approach can also be applied to detect other naturally occurring androgens (DHT), pro-androgens (DHEA and A) or even E administration (attempting to mask T doping by lowering the urine T/E ratio). A limitation of this methodology is the recent identification of a small minority of seized T product samples with nondepleted carbon isotope ratio [83]. The complementary development of hydrogen ion ratio MS further refines the ability to distinguish between endogenous and exogenous steroids in such cases [84, 85].

Another paradigm for detecting androgen abuse is the use of in vitro androgen bioassays [22, 24]. These incorporate the human AR gene together with a convenient AR-mediated response readout indicator into yeast or mammalian cell host cells. Hence, exposure of the host cell to any bioactive androgen will produce a quantifiable signal indicative of androgen bioactivity. These androgen bioassays, aligned with AR activation as the mechanism of androgen doping, provide a generic detection for any bioactive androgen regardless of the chemical structure. While mammalian cells provide a more sensitive host, they also express steroidogenic enzymes and other steroid receptors which thereby sacrifice specificity for sensitivity; however, they also gain the advantage of identifying pro-androgens, chemicals with minimal intrinsic androgen bioactivity but which are converted in the body into potent androgens [24]. By contrast, yeast host cell bioassays display high fidelity in detecting solely intrinsic androgen bioactivity of any chemical, a feature that was crucial in securing the first conviction for use of a designer androgen (tetrahydrogestrinone) previously unknown as an androgen [22]. The detection of any androgen bioactivity provides an advantage over MS, which requires knowledge of the chemical structure of any analyte so, when coupled, they provide powerful additive detection capabilities [86, 87]. Limitations of in vitro androgen bioassays are their susceptibility to nonspecific matrix interference effects from biological fluids such as urine and the difficulty in establishing suitably rigorous standardized methodology involving viable cells. Nevertheless, in vitro androgen bioassays are uniquely useful in screening substances for unsuspected androgenic or pro-androgenic bioactivity [88] which athletes may ingest creating inadvertent doping [57].

Another option to detect androgen doping is the use of hair, skin, or nail samples, which can be minimally invasive, convenient to store dry, and with potentially very long detection windows; however, methodologies have so far been explored only for hair [89–91] and, while used in forensic toxicology, have yet to be accepted for routine anti-doping testing.

Indirect androgen doping involves fewer potential drugs for which detection methods are mostly established. hCG is routinely detected in urine by immunoassays which, unlike LH immunoassay, are validated for human urine having been developed for pregnancy testing and monitoring of trophoblastic tumors [92, 93]. Recently, more accurate, sensitive, and specific immunoextraction-MS proteomic methods are becoming available [94] with some proof-of-principle clinical studies

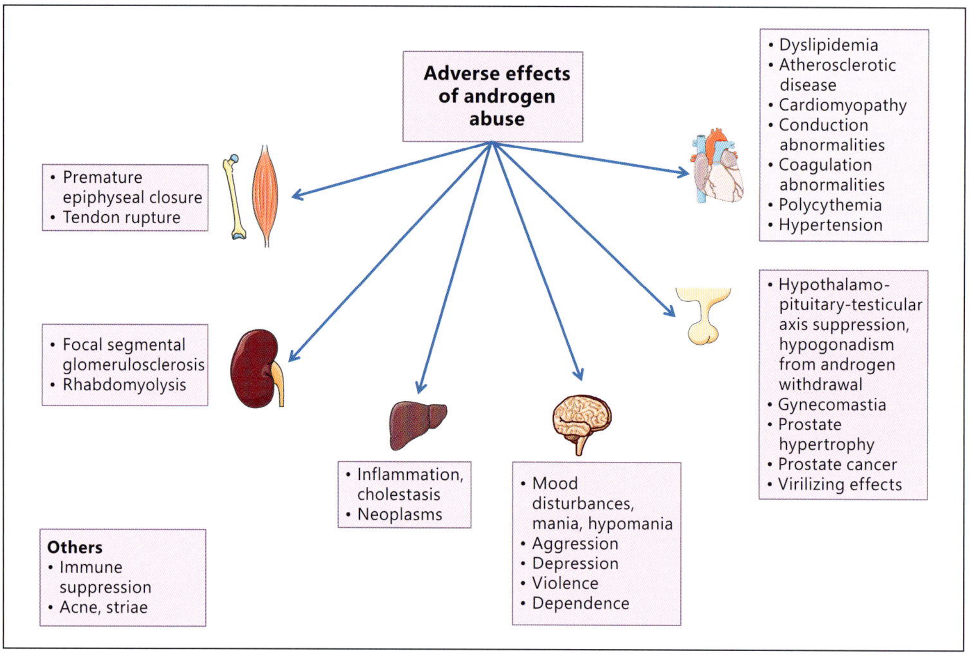

Fig. 2. Common adverse effects of androgen abuse (adverse effect profile adapted from Pope et al. [96]).

[95]. As hCG provides no ergogenic advantage in women, while potentially invading privacy by detecting early pregnancy, hCG testing is confined to men [59]. An important consequence of hCG testing of young male athletes is the detection of early-stage hCG-secreting tumors of the testes or extragonadal midline germ cell tumors which require prompt, expert medical management. Estrogen blockade by anti-estrogens or aromatase inhibitors are routinely included in MS-based urine detection methods.

Adverse Effects of Androgen Abuse

Despite the increasing prevalence of androgen abuse, its adverse effects are not well understood, largely due to its illicit nature leading to underreporting together with very few controlled studies. The adverse effects of androgen abuse have been reviewed in more detail elsewhere [96–98] and so are reviewed here only in outline. They fall into several categories, including cardiovascular, psychological, reproductive, and other effects (fig. 2), but a consistent limitation is the difficulty in establishing causation from observational reports.

A wide variety of cardiovascular harms have been associated with androgen abuse, including cardiomyopathy, myocardial infarction, cardiac tamponade, cardiac failure, arrhythmic sudden death, thrombotic and hemorrhagic stroke, subdural hematoma, peripheral artery and venous thrombosis, and pulmonary embolism; however, the causality of these effects remains speculative and prospective risks difficult to define [97]. A recent randomized, placebo-controlled study of T administration at conventional doses for older men with limited mobility was terminated prematurely due to excess adverse cardiovascular events [99]; however, case-control studies of T administration at conventional doses in older men have produced conflicting findings [100, 101]. It remains suspicious but unproven whether cardiovascular effects of androgen abuse exceed expectations for the general population [102].

Reproductive effects of androgen abuse are profound but at least initially reversible. Suppressing the hypothalamo-pituitary drive to testicular function leads to hypogonadism with consequential testicular atrophy, impaired spermatogenesis, infertility, sexual dysfunction, and gynecomastia. Recovery can be complete but is often slow, with the timing depending on the duration and intensity of preceding androgen abuse. Failure to recover normal testicular function lasting over 1 year is not uncommon, especially among body builders who ingest massive androgen doses without interruption for years. Transient androgen deficiency symptoms may be experienced during prolonged recovery and, while treatment of functional gonadotropin deficiency with hCG or anti-estrogens is possible, ultimately it further delays recovery of the underlying hypothalamic-pituitary suppression. In some cases, apparently prolonged failure to recover may be confused by surreptitious ingestion of androgens during purported recovery.

Hepatotoxicity is a serious adverse effect arising from oral 17α-alkylated androgens but not from other androgens (natural androgens, nandrolone, or 1-methyl androgens) [103]. This includes hepatic tumors (adenoma, carcinoma, cholangiosarcoma, and angiosarcoma) as well as peliosis hepatis and drug hepatotoxicity (usually cholestasis). Most hepatic tumors are slowly progressive and reversible upon cessation of androgen ingestion, but fatal cancers are also reported. Peliosis hepatis, focal hepatic necrosis causing vascular cysts, causes hepatic and/or splenic enlargement and serious, even fatal, bleeding either spontaneously or following liver biopsy.

Adverse psychological disturbances associated with androgen abuse can affect not only the individual but also the community [36]. Mood and behavioral disorders, including hypomania, aggression, depression, and sleep disturbance, are commonly reported by androgen abusers although causality and mechanisms remain speculative. Direct experimental evidence has proven that even a short-term, high-dose androgen exposure may provoke hypomania in apparently healthy volunteers, an idiosyncratic risk affecting an unpredictable small minority (~5%) of individuals [104]. In addition to direct androgen effects, adverse psychological effects may arise from preexisting psychopathology and/or confounding effects of intensive training regimes although parsing these mechanisms is difficult from solely observational evidence. There is increasing evidence that androgen abuse may involve dependence [105] with an undefined relationship to obsessive-compulsive and eating/exercising disorder.

Conclusion

Androgen doping gains ergogenic advantage, is risky to an athlete's health, and is cheating in violation of the spirit of fairness in sport thereby contravening all three WADA Code criteria for prohibition of drugs [43]. In sports, the temptations of cheating to achieve celebrity is enticing not only to elite competitors but also subelite athletes seeking to improve their rank as well as champions whose careers are failing. The highly sensitive urine MS tests for androgens with high risk of detection have driven attempts to exploit alternative forms of androgen doping, such as using unrecognized synthetic designer or nutraceutical androgens or natural androgen, which must be distinguished from their endogenous counterparts. The ongoing challenges to combat androgen doping are to extend the rigorous detection of in-competition to out-of-competition testing both by more random testing during training before competitions as well as the identification of longer-term metabolites that widen the detection window. The goal of deterring drug cheating requires a focus not only on athletes but also on their coaches, who appear to be major determinants of doping susceptibility and practice. Like cybercrime, the continuing rich rewards of androgen doping as potent ergogenic tactic in power sports drives continual development of novel androgen doping threats. This in turn requires ongoing vigilance and inventiveness in anti-doping science to maintain effective deterrence in the face of evolving doping challenges. Outside sports, endemic androgen abuse is indulged in for cosmetic goals such as body sculpting and image enhancement, where the risks are primarily safety of the community as well as the individual abuser. Despite its high prevalence, the current understanding of adverse effects of long-term androgen abuse is based largely on anecdotal evidence. Hence, well-controlled retrospective case-control studies and prospective longitudinal studies of high-risk athletes would be valuable to gain more insight into the safety profile of androgen abuse.

References

1 Handelsman DJ: Androgen physiology, pharmacology and abuse; in DeGroot LJ, Jameson JL (eds): Endocrinology: Adult and Pediatric, ed 7. Philadelphia, Elsevier Saunders, 2015.

2 Li J, Al-Azzawi F: Mechanism of androgen receptor action. Maturitas 2009;63:142–148.

3 Dent JR, Fletcher DK, McGuigan MR: Evidence for a non-genomic action of testosterone in skeletal muscle which may improve athletic performance: implications for the female athlete. J Sports Sci Med 2012;11:363–370.

4 David K, Dingemanse E, Freud J, Laqueur E: Über kristallinisches männliches Hormon aus Hoden (Testosteron), wirksamer als aus Harn oder aus Cholesterin bereitetes Androsteron. Hoppe Seylers Z Physiol Chem 1935;233:281–282.

5 Hamilton JB: Treatment of sexual underdevelopment with synthetic male hormone substance. Endocrinology 1937;21:649–654.

6 Mohler ML, Bohl CE, Jones A, Coss CC, Narayanan R, He Y, Hwang DJ, Dalton JT, Miller DD: Nonsteroidal selective androgen receptor modulators (SARMs): dissociating the anabolic and androgenic activities of the androgen receptor for therapeutic benefit. J Med Chem 2009;52:3597–3617.

7 Hoffman JR, Kraemer WJ, Bhasin S, Storer T, Ratamess NA, Haff GG, Willoughby DS, Rogol AD: Position stand on androgen and human growth hormone use. J Strength Cond Res 2009;23:S1–S59.

8 Handelsman DJ: Commentary: androgens and 'anabolic steroids': the one-headed Janus. Endocrinology 2011;152:1752–1754.
9 Junkman K: Long-acting steroids in reproduction. Recent Prog Horm Res 1957;13:380–419.
10 Kicman AT: Pharmacology of anabolic steroids. Br J Pharmacol 2008;154:502–521.
11 Handelsman DJ: Androgen therapy in non-gonadal disease; in Nieschlag E, Behre HM (eds): Testosterone: Action, Deficiency and Substitution, ed 4. Cambridge, Cambridge University Press, 2011, pp 372–407.
12 Geyer H, Parr MK, Mareck U, Reinhart U, Schrader Y, Schanzer W: Analysis of non-hormonal nutritional supplements for anabolic-androgenic steroids – results of an international study. Int J Sports Med 2004;25:124–129.
13 Thevis M, Geyer H, Thomas A, Schanzer W: Trafficking of drug candidates relevant for sports drug testing: detection of non-approved therapeutics categorized as anabolic and gene doping agents in products distributed via the Internet. Drug Test Anal 2011;3:331–336.
14 Cordaro FG, Lombardo S, Cosentino M: Selling androgenic anabolic steroids by the pound: identification and analysis of popular websites on the Internet. Scand J Med Sci Sports 2011;21:e247–e259.
15 Abbate V, Kicman AT, Evans-Brown M, McVeigh J, Cowan DA, Wilson C, Coles SJ, Walker CJ: Anabolic steroids detected in bodybuilding dietary supplements – a significant risk to public health. Drug Test Anal 2015;7:609–618.
16 Krug O, Thomas A, Walpurgis K, Piper T, Sigmund G, Schanzer W, Laussmann T, Thevis M: Identification of black market products and potential doping agents in Germany 2010–2013. Eur J Clin Pharmacol 2014;70:1303–1311.
17 Rahnema CD, Crosnoe LE, Kim ED: Designer steroids – over-the-counter supplements and their androgenic component: review of an increasing problem. Andrology 2015;3:150–155.
18 Handelsman DJ, Heather A: Androgen abuse in sports. Asian J Androl 2008;10:403–415.
19 Kazlauskas R: Designer steroids (review). Handb Exp Pharmacol 2010;195:155–185.
20 Catlin DH, Ahrens BD, Kucherova Y: Detection of norbolethone, an anabolic steroid never marketed, in athletes' urine. Rapid Commun Mass Spectrom 2002;16:1273–1275.
21 Catlin DH, Sekera MH, Ahrens BD, Starcevic B, Chang YC, Hatton CK: Tetrahydrogestrinone: discovery, synthesis, and detection. Rapid Commun Mass Spectrom 2004;18:1245–1249.
22 Death AK, McGrath KC, Kazlauskas R, Handelsman DJ: Tetrahydrogestrinone is a potent androgen and progestin. J Clin Endocrinol Metab 2004;89:2498–2500.
23 Sekera MH, Ahrens BD, Chang YC, Starcevic B, Georgakopoulos C, Catlin DH: Another designer steroid: discovery, synthesis, and detection of 'Madol' in urine. Rapid Commun Mass Spectrom 2005;19:781–784.
24 Akram ON, Bursill C, Desai R, Heather AK, Kazlauskas R, Handelsman DJ, Lambert G: Evaluation of androgenic activity of nutraceutical-derived steroids using mammalian and yeast in vitro androgen bioassays. Anal Chem 2011;83:2065–2074.
25 Dalton JT, Mukherjee A, Zhu Z, Kirkovsky L, Miller DD: Discovery of nonsteroidal androgens. Biochem Biophys Res Commun 1998;244:1–4.
26 Bhasin S, Jasuja R: Selective androgen receptor modulators as function promoting therapies. Curr Opin Clin Nutr Metab Care 2009;12:232–240.
27 Dobs AS, Boccia RV, Croot CC, Gabrail NY, Dalton JT, Hancock ML, Johnston MA, Steiner MS: Effects of enobosarm on muscle wasting and physical function in patients with cancer: a double-blind, randomised controlled phase 2 trial. Lancet Oncol 2013;14:335–345.
28 Dalton JT, Taylor RP, Mohler ML, Steiner MS: Selective androgen receptor modulators for the prevention and treatment of muscle wasting associated with cancer. Curr Opin Support Palliat Care 2013;7:345–351.
29 Kohler M, Thomas A, Geyer H, Petrou M, Schanzer W, Thevis M: Confiscated black market products and nutritional supplements with non-approved ingredients analyzed in the Cologne Doping Control Laboratory 2009. Drug Test Anal 2010;2:533–537.
30 Grata E, Perrenoud L, Saugy M, Baume N: SARM-S4 and metabolites detection in sports drug testing: a case report. Forensic Sci Int 2011;213:104–108.
31 Starcevic B, Ahrens BD, Butch AW: Detection of the selective androgen receptor modulator S-4 (Andarine) in a doping control sample. Drug Test Anal 2013;5:377–379.
32 Elashoff JD, Jacknow AD, Shain SG, Braunstein GD: Effects of anabolic-androgenic steroids on muscular strength. Ann Intern Med 1991;115:387–393.
33 Bhasin S, Storer TW, Berman N, Callegari C, Clevenger B, Phillips J, Bunnell TJ, Tricker R, Shirazi A, Casaburi R: The effects of supraphysiologic doses of testosterone on muscle size and strength in normal men. N Engl J Med 1996;335:1–7.
34 Handelsman DJ: Performance enhancing hormones in sports doping; in DeGroot LJ, Jameson JL (eds): Endocrinology: Adult and Pediatric, ed 7. Philadelphia, Elsevier Saunders, 2015, pp 441–454.
35 Shahani S, Braga-Basaria M, Maggio M, Basaria S: Androgens and erythropoiesis: past and present. J Endocrinol Invest 2009;32:704–716.
36 Kanayama G, Hudson JI, Pope HG Jr: Long-term psychiatric and medical consequences of anabolic-androgenic steroid abuse: a looming public health concern? Drug Alcohol Depend 2008;98:1–12.

37 Blanco CE, Popper P, Micevych P: Anabolic-androgenic steroid induced alterations in choline acetyltransferase messenger RNA levels of spinal cord motoneurons in the male rat. Neuroscience 1997;78: 873–882.
38 Breedlove SM: Hormonal control of the anatomical specificity of motoneuron-to-muscle innervation in rats. Science 1985;227:1357–1359.
39 Jordan CL, Christensen SE, Handa RJ, Anderson JL, Pouliot WA, Breedlove SM: Evidence that androgen acts through NMDA receptors to affect motoneurons in the rat spinal nucleus of the bulbocavernosus. J Neurosci 2002;22:9567–9572.
40 Franke WW, Berendonk B: Hormonal doping and androgenization of athletes: a secret program of the German Democratic Republic government. Clin Chem 1997;43:1262–1279.
41 Parkinson AB, Evans NA: Anabolic androgenic steroids: a survey of 500 users. Med Sci Sports Exerc 2006;38:644–651.
42 Ip EJ, Barnett MJ, Tenerowicz MJ, Perry PJ: The Anabolic 500 survey: characteristics of male users versus nonusers of anabolic-androgenic steroids for strength training. Pharmacotherapy 2011;31:757–766.
43 WADA: World Anti-Doping Code: 2015. Montreal, WADA, 2015, https://www.wada-ama.org/en/resources/the-code/world-anti-doping-code, https://wada-main-prod.s3.amazonaws.com/resources/files/wada-2015-world-anti-doping-code.pdf.
44 WADA: International Standard. Therapeutic Use Exemptions. Montreal, WADA, 2015, https://wada-main-prod.s3.amazonaws.com/resources/files/WADA-2015-ISTUE-Final-EN.pdf (accessed Oct 2014).
45 WADA: TUE Physician Guidelines. Medical Information to Support the Decisions of TUE Committees – Androgen Deficiency/Male Hypogonadism. Montreal, WADA, 2015, https://wada-main-prod.s3.amazonaws.com/wada-androgen-deficiency-male_hypogonadism-v4.0-en.pdf.
46 WADA: 2013 Anti-Doping Testing Figures – Laboratory Report. Montreal, WADA, 2013, https://wada-main-prod.s3.amazonaws.com/resources/files/WADA-2013-Anti-Doping-Testing-Figures-LABORATORY-REPORT.pdf.
47 Striegel H, Ulrich R, Simon P: Randomized response estimates for doping and illicit drug use in elite athletes. Drug Alcohol Depend 2010;106:230–232.
48 Jalleh G, Donovan RJ, Jobling I: Predicting attitude towards performance enhancing substance use: a comprehensive test of the Sport Drug Control Model with elite Australian athletes. J Sci Med Sport 2014; 17:574–579.
49 Kanayama G, Boynes M, Hudson JI, Field AE, Pope HG Jr: Anabolic steroid abuse among teenage girls: an illusory problem? Drug Alcohol Depend 2007;88: 156–162.
50 Sagoe D, Molde H, Andreassen CS, Torsheim T, Pallesen S: The global epidemiology of anabolic-androgenic steroid use: a meta-analysis and meta-regression analysis. Ann Epidemiol 2014;24:383–398.
51 Buckley WE, Yesalis CE, Freidl KE, Anderson WA, Streit AL, Wright JE: Estimated prevalence of anabolic steroid use among male high school students. JAMA 1988;260:3441–3445.
52 Johnston LD, O'Malley P, Bachman JG, Schulenberg J, Miech R: Monitoring the Future. National Survey Results on Drug Use: 1975–2013. Ann Arbor, Institute for Social Research, University of Michigan, 2014.
53 Pope HG Jr, Kanayama G, Athey A, Ryan E, Hudson JI, Baggish A: The lifetime prevalence of anabolic-androgenic steroid use and dependence in Americans: current best estimates. Am J Addict 2014;23:371–377.
54 Ip EJ, Trinh K, Tenerowicz MJ, Pal J, Lindfelt TA, Perry PJ: Characteristics and behaviors of older male anabolic steroid users. J Pharm Pract 2015;28:450–456.
55 Handelsman DJ, Gupta L: Prevalence and risk factors for anabolic-androgenic steroid abuse in Australian secondary school students. Int J Androl 1997;20:159–164.
56 Baume N, Mahler N, Kamber M, Mangin P, Saugy M: Research of stimulants and anabolic steroids in dietary supplements. Scand J Med Sci Sports 2006; 16:41–48.
57 Geyer H, Schanzer W, Thevis M: Anabolic agents: recent strategies for their detection and protection from inadvertent doping. Br J Sports Med 2014;48: 820–826.
58 Geyer H, Parr MK, Koehler K, Mareck U, Schanzer W, Thevis M: Nutritional supplements cross-contaminated and faked with doping substances. J Mass Spectrom 2008;43:892–902.
59 Handelsman DJ: Clinical review: the rationale for banning human chorionic gonadotropin and estrogen blockers in sport. J Clin Endocrinol Metab 2006; 91:1646–1653.
60 Ayotte C: Detecting the administration of endogenous anabolic androgenic steroids. Handb Exp Pharmacol 2010;195:77–98.
61 Healy DL, Evans J: Creutzfeldt-Jakob disease after pituitary gonadotrophins. BMJ 1993;307:517–518.
62 Liu PY, Baker HW, Jayadev V, Zacharin M, Conway AJ, Handelsman DJ: Induction of spermatogenesis and fertility during gonadotropin treatment of gonadotropin-deficient infertile men: predictors of fertility outcome. J Clin Endocrinol Metab 2009;94: 801–808.

63 Handelsman DJ, Goebel C, Idan A, Jimenez M, Trout G, Kazlauskas R: Effects of recombinant human LH and hCG on serum and urine LH and androgens in men. Clin Endocrinol (Oxf) 2009;71:417–428.
64 Goebel C, Howe CJ, Ho KK, Nelson A, Kazlauskas R, Trout GJ: Screening for testosterone abuse in male athletes using the measurement of urinary LH, a revision of the paradigm. Drug Test Anal 2009;1:511–517.
65 Maximov PY, Lee TM, Jordan VC: The discovery and development of selective estrogen receptor modulators (SERMs) for clinical practice. Curr Clin Pharmacol 2013;8:135–155.
66 Santen RJ, Brodie H, Simpson ER, Siiteri PK, Brodie A: History of aromatase: saga of an important biological mediator and therapeutic target. Endocr Rev 2009;30:343–375.
67 Handelsman DJ: Indirect androgen doping by oestrogen blockade in sports. Br J Pharmacol 2008;154: 598–605.
68 Perry PJ, Lund BC, Deninger MJ, Kutscher EC, Schneider J: Anabolic steroid use in weightlifters and bodybuilders: an internet survey of drug utilization. Clin J Sport Med 2005;15:326–330.
69 Hall RC, Hall RC: Abuse of supraphysiologic doses of anabolic steroids. South Med J 2005;98:550–555.
70 Sheffield-Moore M, Dillon EL, Casperson SL, Gilkison CR, Paddon-Jones D, Durham WJ, Grady JJ, Urban RJ: A randomized pilot study of monthly cycled testosterone replacement or continuous testosterone replacement versus placebo in older men. J Clin Endocrinol Metab 2011;96:E1831–E1837.
71 Fitts RH, Peters JR, Dillon EL, Durham WJ, Sheffield-Moore M, Urban RJ: Weekly versus monthly testosterone administration on fast and slow skeletal muscle fibers in older adult males. J Clin Endocrinol Metab 2015;100:E223–E231.
72 Goldberg L, Elliot DL, Clarke GN, MacKinnon DP, Moe E, Zoref L, Green C, Wolf SL, Greffath E, Miller DJ, Lapin A: Effects of a multidimensional anabolic steroid prevention intervention: the Adolescents Training and Learning to Avoid Steroids (ATLAS) program. JAMA 1996;276:1555–1562.
73 Morente-Sanchez J, Zabala M: Doping in sport: a review of elite athletes' attitudes, beliefs, and knowledge. Sports Med 2013;43:395–411.
74 Guddat S, Fussholler G, Beuck S, Thomas A, Geyer H, Rydevik A, Bondesson U, Hedeland M, Lagojda A, Schanzer W, Thevis M: Synthesis, characterization, and detection of new oxandrolone metabolites as long-term markers in sports drug testing. Anal Bioanal Chem 2013;405:8285–8294.
75 Schanzer W, Guddat S, Thomas A, Opfermann G, Geyer H, Thevis M: Expanding analytical possibilities concerning the detection of stanozolol misuse by means of high resolution/high accuracy mass spectrometric detection of stanozolol glucuronides in human sports drug testing. Drug Test Anal 2013;5: 810–818.
76 Balcells G, Pozo OJ, Esquivel A, Kotronoulas A, Joglar J, Segura J, Ventura R: Screening for anabolic steroids in sports: analytical strategy based on the detection of phase I and phase II intact urinary metabolites by liquid chromatography tandem mass spectrometry. J Chromatogr A 2015;1389:65–75.
77 Xue Y, Sun D, Daly A, Yang F, Zhou X, Zhao M, Huang N, Zerjal T, Lee C, Carter NP, Hurles ME, Tyler-Smith C: Adaptive evolution of UGT2B17 copy-number variation. Am J Hum Genet 2008;83: 337–346.
78 Schulze JJ, Lundmark J, Garle M, Skilving I, Ekstrom L, Rane A: Doping test results dependent on genotype of uridine diphospho-glucuronosyl transferase 2B17, the major enzyme for testosterone glucuronidation. J Clin Endocrinol Metab 2008;93:2500–2506.
79 Vernec AR: The Athlete Biological Passport: an integral element of innovative strategies in antidoping. Br J Sports Med 2014;48:817–819.
80 Sottas PE, Saudan C, Schweizer C, Baume N, Mangin P, Saugy M: From population- to subject-based limits of T/E ratio to detect testosterone abuse in elite sports. Forensic Sci Int 2008;174:166–172.
81 Perry PJ, MacIndoe JH, Yates WR, Scott SD, Holman TL: Detection of anabolic steroid administration: ratio of urinary testosterone to epitestosterone vs the ratio of urinary testosterone to luteinizing hormone. Clin Chem 1997;43:731–735.
82 Singh GK, Jimenez M, Newman R, Handelsman DJ: Immunoreactive LH in long-term frozen human urine samples. Drug Test Anal 2014;6:336–341.
83 Cawley A, Collins M, Kazlauskas R, Handelsman DJ, Heywood R, Longworth M, Arenas-Queralt A: Stable isotope ratio profiling of testosterone preparations. Drug Test Anal 2010;2:557–567.
84 Piper T, Emery C, Thomas A, Saugy M, Thevis M: Combination of carbon isotope ratio with hydrogen isotope ratio determinations in sports drug testing. Anal Bioanal Chem 2013;405:5455–5466.
85 Piper T, Thomas A, Thevis M, Saugy M: Investigations on hydrogen isotope ratios of endogenous urinary steroids: reference-population-based thresholds and proof-of-concept. Drug Test Anal 2012;4: 717–727.
86 Nielen MW, Bovee TF, van Engelen MC, Rutgers P, Hamers AR, van Rhijn JH, Hoogenboom LR: Urine testing for designer steroids by liquid chromatography with androgen bioassay detection and electrospray quadrupole time-of-flight mass spectrometry identification. Anal Chem 2006;78:424–431.

87 Bauer A, Rataj F, Zierau O, Anielski P, Grosse J, Parr MK, Vollmer G, Thieme D: Characterization of identity, metabolism and androgenic activity of 17-hydroxyandrosta-3,5-diene by GC-MS and a yeast transactivation system. Arch Toxicol 2012;86:1873–1884.
88 McRobb L, Handelsman DJ, Kazlauskas R, Wilkinson S, McLeod MD, Heather AK: Structure-activity relationships of synthetic progestins in a yeast-based in vitro androgen bioassay. J Steroid Biochem Mol Biol 2008;110:39–47.
89 Deshmukh N, Hussain I, Barker J, Petroczi A, Naughton DP: Analysis of anabolic steroids in human hair using LC-MS/MS. Steroids 2010;75:710–714.
90 Deshmukh NI, Barker J, Petroczi A, Naughton DP: Detection of testosterone and epitestosterone in human hair using liquid chromatography-tandem mass spectrometry. J Pharm Biomed Anal 2012;67–68:154–158.
91 Kintz P: Testing for anabolic steroids in hair: a review. Leg Med (Tokyo) 2003;5(suppl 1):S29–S33.
92 Stenman UH, Hotakainen K, Alfthan H: Gonadotropins in doping: pharmacological basis and detection of illicit use. Br J Pharmacol 2008;154:569–583.
93 Kuuranne T, Ahola L, Pussinen C, Leinonen A: Analysis of human chorionic gonadotropin (hCG): application of routine immunological methods for initial testing and confirmation analysis in doping control. Drug Test Anal 2013;5:614–618.
94 Woldemariam GA, Butch AW: Immunoextraction-tandem mass spectrometry method for measuring intact human chorionic gonadotropin, free beta-subunit, and beta-subunit core fragment in urine. Clin Chem 2014;60:1089–1097.
95 Lund H, Snilsberg AH, Paus E, Halvorsen TG, Hemmersbach P, Reubsaet L: Sports drug testing using immuno-MS: clinical study comprising administration of human chorionic gonadotropin to males. Anal Bioanal Chem 2013;405:1569–1576.
96 Pope HG Jr, Wood R, Rogol A, Nyberg F, Bowers L, Bhasin S: Adverse health consequences of performance-enhancing drugs: an Endocrine Society scientific statement. Endocr Rev 2014;35:341–375.
97 Vanberg P, Atar D: Androgenic anabolic steroid abuse and the cardiovascular system. Handb Exp Pharmacol 2010;195:411–457.
98 Handelsman DJ: Androgen misuse and abuse. Best Pract Res Clin Endocrinol Metab 2011;25:377–389.
99 Bachman E, Feng R, Travison T, Li M, Olbina G, Ostland V, Ulloor J, Zhang A, Basaria S, Ganz T, Westerman M, Bhasin S: Testosterone suppresses hepcidin in men: a potential mechanism for testosterone-induced erythrocytosis. J Clin Endocrinol Metab 2010;95:4743–4747.
100 Xu L, Freeman G, Cowling BJ, Schooling CM: Testosterone therapy and cardiovascular events among men: a systematic review and meta-analysis of placebo-controlled randomized trials. BMC Med 2013;11:108.
101 Ruige JB, Ouwens DM, Kaufman JM: Beneficial and adverse effects of testosterone on the cardiovascular system in men. J Clin Endocrinol Metab 2013;98:4300–4310.
102 Liu PY, Death AK, Handelsman DJ: Androgens and cardiovascular disease. Endocr Rev 2003;24:313–340.
103 Ishak KG, Zimmerman HJ: Hepatotoxic effects of the anabolic-androgenic steroids. Semin Liver Dis 1987;7:230–236.
104 Pope HG Jr, Kouri EM, Hudson JI: Effects of supraphysiologic doses of testosterone on mood and aggression in normal men: a randomized controlled trial. Arch Gen Psychiatry 2000;57:133–140; discussion 155–136.
105 Kanayama G, Brower KJ, Wood RI, Hudson JI, Pope HG Jr: Anabolic-androgenic steroid dependence: an emerging disorder. Addiction 2009;104:1966–1978.

Prof. David J. Handelsman
ANZAC Research Institute
Sydney, NSW 2139 (Australia)
E-Mail djh@anzac.edu.au

Lanfranco F, Strasburger CJ (eds): Sports Endocrinology.
Front Horm Res. Basel, Karger, 2016, vol 47, pp 101–114 (DOI: 10.1159/000445173)

Growth Hormone and Insulin-Like Growth Factor-1

Adam R. Nicholls • Richard I.G. Holt

Human Development and Health Academic Unit, Faculty of Medicine, University of Southampton, Southampton, UK

Abstract

Human growth hormone (GH) was first isolated from the human pituitary gland in 1945 and found to promote the growth of children with hypopituitarism. Since the formation of the World Anti-Doping Association, human GH has appeared on the list of forbidden substances. There is a significant amount of anecdotal evidence that human GH is misused by athletes to enhance performance, and there have been a number of high-profile cases of GH use in professional sport. GH secretagogues (GH-Ss), which increase GH secretion, and insulin-like growth factor (IGF-1), which mediates many of the effects of GH, are also misused, although there is less evidence for this. The effectiveness of GH, IGF-1, and GH-Ss as performance-enhancing drugs remains unclear. Evidence from studies of GH use in people with hypopituitarism show several desirable outcomes, including increased lean body mass, increased strength, and increased exercise capacity. These anabolic and metabolic properties, coupled with the difficulty in detecting them, make them attractive as agents of misuse. Studies in healthy young adults have also demonstrated a performance benefit with GH and IGF-1.

Human growth hormone (hGH) is a naturally occurring peptide hormone secreted by the anterior pituitary gland. It was first extracted from the human pituitary in 1945 and was shown to promote growth in children with hypopituitarism [1]. Since the formation of the World Anti-Doping Association (WADA) in 1999, hGH has always featured on its list of prohibited substances and appears in the same category as insulin [2]. Prior to this, hGH was included in the International Olympic Committee's list

Table 1. The physiological effects of GH and IGF-1

	Actions of GH	Actions of IGF-1
Body composition	Decreases fat mass Increases lean body mass Increases bone mineral density	Conflicting evidence – may have similar effects to GH
Physical performance	Increases muscle mass and strength Increases VO_{2max}, maximal heart rate, and maximal power output	Increased VO_{2max} Anabolic effect on respiratory muscles
Cardiovascular changes	Increases left-ventricular mass with corresponding increase in stroke volume and cardiac output	Regulation of vascular tone Levels correlate with haemoglobin so may increase oxygen delivery
Intermediate metabolism		
Glucose	Induces peripheral insulin resistance Reduces skeletal muscle glucose uptake	Increases peripheral insulin sensitivity in skeletal muscle and adipose tissue
Fat	Lipolysis – causing increased availability of free fatty acids	GH effects on fat metabolism are independent of IGF-1
Protein	Increased protein synthesis	Increased protein synthesis
Bone	Increases longitudinal bone growth Increases bone mineral density	Increases longitudinal bone growth

of forbidden compounds, once it became clear that more advanced technology made its production easier and, therefore, more available [3].

It is unclear for how long and to what extent it has been used as a performance-enhancing substance by athletes, but one of the most famous cases dates back to 1988 when Ben Johnson admitted misusing GH in addition to anabolic steroids following his disqualification after he had won the gold medal in the 100 m at the Seoul Olympic games [1, 4]. Notably, this predates the use of GH by adult endocrinologists to treat adult GH deficiency by about a decade.

GH has a number of properties that are attractive to athletes wishing to improve their performance (table 1), but it is mainly misused because of its anabolic and lipolytic properties. GH administration leads to increased muscle mass and a decrease in and redistribution of body fat from central to peripheral depots, thereby potentially improving the power-to-weight ratio of an athlete. Despite this theoretical benefit, it is unclear how effective these changes are in improving performance amongst professional athletes [2].

Until recently, a lack of effective anti-doping tests for GH may have encouraged athletes to misuse GH rather than other performance-enhancing drugs, such as androgenic anabolic steroids. In the last decade, WADA has introduced the isoform and GH-2000 biomarker tests to detect GH misuse, and so the pattern of misuse may change; there are already anecdotes that athletes are turning to insulin-like growth factor (IGF)-1 and GH secretagogues (GH-Ss) as alternatives [5].

This chapter will describe the history of GH misuse and will explain the physiological actions that may lead to improved performance. It will consider the evidence to support a performance benefit in young healthy adults. The effects of GH will be compared and contrasted with those of GH-S and IGF-1.

The Misuse of Growth Hormone, Insulin-Like Growth Factor-1, and Growth Hormone Secretagogues in Sport

The role and physiology of GH first became apparent in 1909 when Harvey Cushing identified the aetiology of acromegaly. GH has been used as a performance-enhancing agent since at latest the early 1980s when its use was clearly documented in the *Underground Steroid Handbook* written in 1982 by Dan Duchaine [6]. This magazine was a practical guide to steroid use – indeed, the author admitted it was written under the influence of a large dose of testosterone – but included a chapter on human GH advocating its use to improve performance. One of its claims was that hGH strengthens tendons and reduces the injury that can be caused during powerlifting. Interestingly, these claims were later refuted in the 2nd edition of the *Underground Steroid Handbook*, when the author admitted the original claims were anecdotal and proposed that misuse of hGH was not an effective way of improving performance.

hGH misuse in sport predates its use in adult endocrinology by 10 years, although cadaveric GH had been used in children from the 1950s. This practice was stopped by clinicians (but not athletes) when cases of Creutzfeldt-Jakob disease were discovered in patients who had previously received hGH. The clinical use of GH resumed following the US Food and Drug Agency (FDA) approval of the first synthetic recombinant human (rh)GH, Protropin, in 1985. Other formulations subsequently followed [5].

Evidence of the extent or duration of misuse of hGH in athletes is scarce although, following the confession of Ben Johnson, there has been a steady stream of athletes who have confessed to or have been caught taking GH (table 2). At the Sydney 2000 Olympic Games, the media reported a large targeted theft of hGH from a Sydney importer, which was never recovered. There have been accusations of hGH doping within Major League Baseball, as noted in the Mitchell [7] report, and the National Football League. As described in the book *Game of Shadows*, two journalists from San Francisco discovered that the Bay Area Laboratory Cooperative was supplying performance-enhancing drugs, including GH, to athletes, including the British sprinters Dwaine Chambers and Marion Jones, the five-time track and field Olympic medal winner, who subsequently served a-6 month jail sentence for lying about this misuse [8].

Table 2. Chronology of GH, IGF-1, and GH-S doping in sport

Date	Clinical	Doping
GH doping		
1945	GH extracted	
1955	GH used to treat hypopituitary patients	
1965		
1975	rhGH introduced	Publication of the *Underground Steroid Handbook*
1985	Trials show benefit of GH in adults	Ben Johnson admits taking GH at the Seoul Olympics
1995	GH licensed for use in adult GH deficiency	Atlanta 'GH Games'
		Yuan Yuan (swimmer) smuggles GH during the world championship into Australia
		GH found at the Tour de France
		Werner Reiterer alleges systemic GH doping
2005		BALCO scandal
		Publication of the Mitchell [7] report – an investigation into performance-enhancing drug use in Major League Baseball
		Dwain Chambers admits using GH
		Terry Newton (Rugby League) is the first sportsman to test positive with the isoform detection method
		Andrus Veerpalu tests positive but is later acquitted by the Court of Arbitration for Sport
		Inna Eftimova is the first female track athlete to test positive for GH
		Andreas Klier admits the use of GH during his cycling career claiming endemic use in the sport
		Nikolay Marfin and Vadim Rkatitin (Russian powerlifters) test positive using the GH-2000 biomarker test at the London 2012 Olympics
2015		James Lockwood (Rugby League) tests positive for GHRP-2

Following the introduction of the GH isoform test in 2004, the rugby league player Terry Newton became the first sportsman to be banned following an adverse analytical test finding in 2010 [9]. Since then, further athletes have been detected taking hGH in a range of sports, including swimming, athletics, skiing, powerlifting, cycling, American football and baseball. There were also adverse analytical test findings that led to the suspension of two powerlifters at the 2012 London Paralympic Games 6 weeks following the introduction of the GH-2000 biomarker test. These athletes are likely to represent the minority given the large amount of anecdotal evidence of GH misuse [10].

The Misuse of Insulin-Like Growth Factor-1 in Sport

IGF-1, which also appears on the WADA list of prohibited substances, is thought to mediate many of the anabolic effects of GH, as well as acting as a circulating marker of GH action. Although much less common because of its lack of availability, there is anecdotal evidence that IGF-1 misuse, either alone or in combination with GH, has been increasing for several years. rhIGF-1 has only recently been approved for use in humans (to treat children with certain forms of short stature), and its increased availability is likely to increase its misuse.

The Misuse of Growth Hormone Secretagogues in Sport

GH-Ss are small synthetic peptide and non-peptide molecules that stimulate GH release from the pituitary in a dose-dependent fashion. The endogenous GH-S receptor, which was cloned in 1996, is widely expressed throughout the body, notably within the pancreas and heart, and at high density in the pituitary and hypothalamus [11]. Activation of the GH-S receptor increases the amplitude of GH pulsatility and reduces the somatostatin-inhibitory action on the release of GH from somatotrophs [12]. In 1999, ghrelin, the endogenous ligand of the GH-S receptor, was discovered. Ghrelin is a potent stimulator of GH release acting in a dose-dependent fashion.

GH-releasing peptides (GHRPs) are a heterogeneous group which makes them an appealing agent for doping. Although GHRPs can be detected directly, the large number of peptides makes it challenging to detect all of these compounds [13]. Nevertheless at least one athlete has been detected in this manner. GHRPs are potent stimulators of GH release and so may have similar benefits to misusing hGH [12]. The use of synthetic GH-S (MK-0677) in older people restores GH secretion to that of young adults and has been shown to increase lean body mass, increase bone mineral density, and lead to a modest increase in strength [12].

The Growth Hormone Axis and Growth Hormone Physiology

GH is secreted from somatotroph cells of the anterior pituitary gland under the influence of both central and peripheral mechanisms. Its release is under direct control of two principal hypothalamic hormones, GH-releasing hormone (GHRH), which promotes secretion, and somatostatin, which inhibits it [14]. GHRH and somatostatin secretion is modulated by a number of other factors, including catecholamines and steroid hormones (table 3). GH secretion is also increased by ghrelin, which is

Table 3. Factors influencing GH release

Stimulates GH release	
Peptide hormones	
	GHRH
	Ghrelin
Sex hormones	
	Increased androgen secretion during puberty
	Estrogen
Stimulation of GHRH release	
	Clonidine
	L-DOPA
	$\alpha_4\beta_2$ nicotinic agonists (including nicotine)
Inhibition of somatostatin release	
	Hypoglycaemia
	Arginine
	Propranolol
Miscellaneous	
	Nicotinic acid
	Vigorous exercise
	Deep sleep
Inhibits GH release	
Peptide hormones	
	Somatostatin
	IGF-1
Steroid hormones	
	Glucocorticoids
	Dihydrotestosterone
Miscellaneous	
	Hyperglycaemia

produced in the gastrointestinal tract [15]. A number of other endogenous GHRPs have been described. In addition to stimulation of GH release, GHRPs cause varying increases in prolactin and adrenocorticotropic hormone (ACTH) [16].

GH is secreted in a pulsatile fashion in 6–8 bursts per day, with negligible secretion between these times. There is a large pulse at the onset of slow-wave sleep, and smaller pulses several hours after meals [17, 18].

The majority of circulating GH is bound to GH binding protein, which corresponds to the extracellular part of the GH receptor, with only 20% of plasma GH being in its monomeric form. GH exerts its actions through binding to two cell surface receptors. Intra-cellular signalling pathways result in the activation of transcription factors on targeted genes, for example the gene promoter region on the IGF-1 gene resulting in increased IGF-1 production [18].

GH promotes IGF-1 secretion, predominantly from the liver, which in turn circulates in the blood and feeds back to the hypothalamus to inhibit GH secretion. GH also feeds back to the hypothalamus itself thereby reducing the pulsatile secretion of further GH [17]. There is an age-related decline in GH levels which may relate to decreasing levels of GHRH levels and increasing somatostatin tone [17].

GH can exert both IGF-1-dependent and IGF-1-independent actions, but it is thought that IGF-1-independent actions predominate in the fasted state, when GH levels are at their highest [14, 18]. Overall GH and IGF-1 act in a coordinated manner with insulin to promote growth at times of sufficient nutrient supply by enabling cell hypertrophy in response to the correct stimulus, to prevent apoptosis, and to enable cell division. In addition, both hormones have important metabolic effects [19].

Effects of Growth Hormone and Insulin-Like Growth Factor-1 on Lipid Metabolism
The effects of GH on lipid metabolism are most marked overnight, corresponding to the large surge in GH levels at the onset of slow-wave sleep [14]. GH stimulates lipolysis in abdominal fat [18], and this is associated with rising free fatty acids and glycerol, and increased production of ketone bodies. As this mainly happens at night, it is likely that the physiological role is to switch energy production from glucose and protein metabolism to fat metabolism in the fasted state. Long-term GH treatment is associated with increased lean body mass and decreased visceral fat.

GH affects hepatic lipid metabolism most notably by increasing lipoprotein lipase activity and increased intra-hepatic triglyceride storage while suppressing intra-hepatic lipolysis. Many of its effects are exerted in an IGF-1-independent manner [15]. GH has a similar effect on lipid storage in skeletal muscles as people with acromegaly, and adults treated for GH deficiency have increased myocellular triglyceride levels. Lipolysis and lipid oxidation are increased in skeletal muscles in the presence of GH. It may be that this action is context dependent, for example, during exercise or during a period of fasting [15]. This may be one of the reasons why skeletal muscle fat metabolism increases during periods of prolonged exercise, corresponding to the increased GH seen at this time.

Effects of Growth Hormone and Insulin-Like Growth Factor-1 on Insulin and Carbohydrate Metabolism
The effects of GH on glucose metabolism are complex [15]. An acute peripheral intravenous infusion of GH decreases muscle glucose uptake, induces a state of peripheral insulin resistance, and leads to increased utilization of fat as a fuel substrate in muscles [20]. If GH is deficient or removed for a short period of time, there is a state of increased insulin sensitivity; however, long-term changes in body composition (as discussed later) lead to increased insulin resistance. One may assume that reduced skeletal muscle glucose uptake would lead to increased plasma glucose, but this is not the case because increased glucose uptake and diminished gluconeogenesis may occur within the liver or kidney in the presence of elevated GH levels [20]. The increase in free fatty acids as a result of the lipolytic action of GH may further reduce the action of insulin on target tissues [15]. This reduces the dependence on glucose as a fuel source, which may be beneficial during exercise.

IGF-1 has structural homology to insulin and binds to the insulin receptor, albeit with low affinity and a glucose-lowering ability that is one twelfth that of insulin. Consequently, GH and IGF-1 have opposing effects on insulin sensitivity, and this is likely to exert differential effects in different tissues. GH reduces insulin suppression of hepatic gluconeogenesis while IGF-1 increases insulin sensitivity peripherally in skeletal muscles and adipose tissue, and negatively feeds back to lower GH concentration [21]. Again, this balance between GH and IGF-1 may be important in the partition of nutrients during times of starvation and adequate nutrition. This complex interaction will also have an important role in fuel metabolism during exercise.

Effects of Growth Hormone and Insulin-Like Growth Factor-1 on Protein Metabolism
GH exerts a net anabolic effect on protein metabolism either directly or via IGF-1 [17]. IGF-1-driven protein synthesis is reduced by AMP kinase, which is activated by nutrient restriction and exercise. This supports the theory that IGF-1 is important for growth in times of adequate nutrition. Insulin and IGF-1 have some synergistic actions in maintaining protein balance. Insulin decreases proteolysis within muscles at very low concentrations and so is probably the most important factor in protein balance following a meal containing adequate calories [19]. This is particularly relevant to exercise in times of both recovery from injury and increasing lean body mass.

Effect of Growth Hormone and Insulin-Like Growth Factor-1 on Cortisol
GH has a modulatory effect on 11β-hydroxylase, which converts cortisone to active cortisol. Consequently, in the absence of GH, increased 11β-hydroxylase activity leads to increased visceral availability of cortisol thereby driving the increased visceral fat seen in GH deficiency and cortisol excess. However, in people with intact ACTH, any fall in peripheral cortisol by exposure to increased GH is matched by increased ACTH secretion, maintaining normal cortisol concentrations. The interaction between GH and cortisol may have a role to play when considering GH misuse and altered fat distribution, as reduction in visceral fat combined with the lipolytic action of GH may seem attractive to athletes wishing to misuse GH [22].

Effects of Growth Hormone and Insulin-Like Growth Factor-1 on Bone
GH and IGF-1 are important regulators of bone and soft tissue growth, and GH is thought to be one of the key determinants of adult bone mass. The effects of IGF-1 and GH on bone are different, but synergistic. GH has a stimulatory effect on both collagen and bone, as noted by increases in biomarkers of collagen growth and markers of bone turnover following GH administration [23, 24].

In animal models, IGF-1 stimulates pre-chondrocytes at a later stage of development than GH. The administration of IGF-1 alone results in increased longitudinal bone growth, an effect that lessens with time. The addition of GH results in increased growth.

GH has a positive effect on bone mineral density in post-menopausal women and improves functional outcomes, such as muscle strength, following hip fracture. GH levels are known to decrease with age, and the greatest benefit is purported to occur in older, frailer individuals [25, 26].

In human studies of osteoporosis, IGF-1 levels are lower in post-menopausal women and men with osteoporosis although the results of studies of IGF-1 treatment in osteoporosis are inconclusive, mainly because of the sample size of these studies [24].

It is difficult to be certain from animal studies whether the effects of GH on bone are mediated by the endocrine effects of IGF-1 or whether IGF-1 has an independent autocrine or paracrine effect on bone. However, experimental studies have demonstrated that mice with IGF-1 gene deletions have severe growth retardation, and that IGF-1 also stimulates longitudinal bone growth in hypophysectomised rats [23, 24].

Despite a lack of evidence, this potential effect of GH on the growth of bone and soft tissue has been proposed as a means of aiding healing in athletes – a fact attributed to it by the *Underground Steroid Handbook* [10]. This is supported by long-term studies of GH treatment in adults with GH deficiency which demonstrated beneficial changes in bone mineral density after 10 years of treatment [27, 28].

Growth Hormone in Sports and Performance

Although the actions of GH and IGF-1 described in the previous section offer reasons why athletes may misuse GH, the question remains whether it improves athletic performance [5, 29, 30].

The Effect of Growth Hormone and Insulin-Like Growth Factor-1 on Body Composition

The effects of GH on adult body composition were first studied in people with GH deficiency. Following GH treatment, there was a marked sustained reduction in total body fat, which was accompanied by a similar increase in lean body mass [19]. Studies of people with obesity have shown that IGF-1 concentration is reduced, while GH supplementation in older obese individuals led to a small reduction in visceral fat [31]. There appears to be a synergistic effect with testosterone as older men receiving both hormones had a larger increase in lean body mass than those receiving GH or testosterone alone [32]. The enhanced effect of testosterone supplementation with GH was one of the perceived benefits of GH claimed in the *Underground Steroid Handbook*, and this has been a research focus in age-related sarcopenia and obesity [27, 28].

Increased lean body mass and decreased fat mass have also been seen in young adults who have received GH. A recent systematic review of 44 articles describing 27 study samples including 303 participants found a 2.1-kg increase in lean body mass and 0.9-kg decrease in fat mass [33].

There have been conflicting reports of the effects of IGF-1 administration on body composition, depending on the population studied. In a group of obese post-menopausal women, the administration of rhGH alone and rhGH combined with rhIGF-1 led to increased fat-free mass, but rhIGF alone had no effect [34]. rhIGF-1 administration was associated with increased lean body mass and decreased adiposity in adults with GH deficiency [35] or GH insensitivity syndrome [22]. These changes were attributed to the stimulatory effects of rhIGF-1 on lipolysis and lipid oxidation in adults with GH insensitivity syndrome. However, no changes in lean body mass or adipose tissue were observed after rhIGF-1 was administered to healthy post-menopausal women or recreational athletes [36].

The Effect of Exercise on Growth Hormone and Insulin-Like Growth Factor-1

Exercise is the most potent physiological stimulus for GH release. GH starts to rise within 10–20 min of commencing exercise and peaks at the end or shortly after completion [29]. A number of factors affect the increase in GH, including age, gender, body composition, intensity, and duration of exercise. Exercise increases the amplitude of each GH pulse rather than the frequency. Studies assessing total and free levels of IGF-1 have been conflicting, with some showing an increase, some showing a decrease, but most showing no change in free IGF-1 [29]. These differences probably relate to the study design and participants, but it seems unlikely that GH exerts its effects during exercise through increases in IGF-1. This is in contrast to studies of GH administration at supra-physiological doses, which reported increases in circulating IGF-1 [30].

The physiological relevance of the GH peak after exercise is uncertain but may increase protein synthesis and aid in muscle repair after exercise. The increase in muscle triglycerides may also be important in preventing hypoglycemia following exercise by promoting free fatty acids as an energy substrate at a time when carbohydrate stores are predicted to be low [29, 33].

The Effect of Growth Hormone and Insulin-Like Growth Factor-1 Administration on Exercise Performance

Although there is incontrovertible evidence that GH leads to changes in body composition, evidence is only just emerging that it improves exercise performance in healthy young adults. During exercise, metabolic fuels, such as glucose for short-term, high-intensity activity and free fatty acids for more prolonged activity, are combusted to release kinetic energy. Thus, performance depends on the availability of metabolic fuels and oxygen in exercising muscles and GH may improve performance through increased delivery of fuels and oxygen, increased muscle strength, or any combination of these factors.

The first studies on performance come from the treatment of adults with GH deficiency. The early studies used GH doses that would now be considered supra-physiological. Nevertheless, these showed that GH improved VO_{2max} (aerobic capacity, the maximum ability to take in and use oxygen) and the maximum work rate [37]. The magnitude of the increase in VO_{2max} was proportional to the gain in lean body mass. When VO_{2max} is low, the lactate threshold is reached at lower exercise intensity or duration causing early fatigue and reduced exercise capability [29, 37]. Increases in VO_{2max} and the lactate threshold are seen with athletic training [17]. The observed proportional increase in VO_{2max} and lean body mass in individuals treated with GH may explain the reduction in fatigue and improved exercise seen in the studies [33].

GH increases plasma volume and subsequently pre-load and stroke volume which may lead to increased cardiac output. There is also evidence that GH has a positive effect on left-ventricular ejection fraction. All of these factors may improve exercise capability [29].

Whether these effects in elderly adults can be extrapolated to young adults is debatable because of the major differences in GH secretion between the young and the old. This is supported by a systematic review of 303 participants that found no effect of GH on the respiratory quotient, VO_{2max}, bicycling speed, power output, energy expenditure, or strength [33].

These findings, however, have been challenged more recently by two studies; the first was conducted in a cohort of ex-anabolic steroid abusers administered rhGH for 6 days [38]. In addition to the expected body composition changes, strength and peak power output significantly increased. It is possible that this study found a performance benefit because the athletes may have been particularly sensitive to the anabolic actions of GH due to their prior use of steroids. The second study demonstrated a short-lived increase in sprint capacity in both men and women, with a synergistic effect of testosterone in men, which had disappeared 6 weeks after GH discontinuation [39].

Very few studies have been undertaken to examine the effects of IGF-1 on performance, but we have recently demonstrated a 9% increase in VO_{2max} in recreational athletes following a 28-day administration of rhIGF-1/rhIGF binding protein-3 despite no change in body composition [36]. The mechanism underlying this change is unknown, but previous studies have shown that the intravenous administration of rhIGF-1 caused an increase in cardiac output, heart rate, and stroke volume in healthy adults [18]. IGF-1 may have a role in the regulation of vascular tone through alterations in nitric oxide synthesis [19], allowing improved intramuscular blood flow. Serum IGF-1 correlates positively with hemoglobin concentration, which may enhance oxygen delivery to exercising muscle. Finally, an anabolic effect on respiratory muscle strength may improve inspiratory effort.

There are no published studies of the effects of GH-Ss on performance, but studies have shown that these increase GH secretion and potentially could improve athleticism through this mechanism. Given the difficulties in demonstrating an effect of GH, even at supra-physiological doses, it seems unlikely that we will have definitive proof of a performance effect for GH-Ss in the near future.

Potential Adverse Effects of Administration

Poison is in everything, and no thing is without poison.
The dosage makes it either a poison or a remedy.
Paracelsus

While there may be performance benefits, the administration of GH, IGF-1, or GH-S may also place the athlete at risk of harm. The side effects of GH administration in the treatment of GH deficiency are well documented and may affect any athlete taking GH [40]; however, it is reported that some athletes are using doses that are up to 10-fold higher than the therapeutic doses. The long-term effects of GH administration may, therefore, include fluid retention, leading to ankle swelling, hypertension, headache, diabetes, and cardiomyopathy, which is characterized by abnormalities in cardiac muscle structure and function. The risk of certain cancers, including colorectal, thyroid, breast, and prostate cancer, may be increased, but this is controversial [41].

Although all pharmaceutically available rhGH is now manufactured using recombinant DNA technology, some athletes continue to use supplies of pituitary-derived GH that are still available on the black market, thereby putting themselves at risk of the prion-induced Creutzfeldt-Jakob disease [42].

There are many reported side effects of IGF-1 administration, particularly at supra-physiological doses: hypoglycaemia, oedema, headache, syncope, arthralgia, jaw pain, and breathlessness [43].

Conclusion

There is ample evidence that GH, and more recently IGF-1 and GH-S, have been misused by athletes wishing to improve their performance. The advent of improved detection methods has highlighted a number of athletes who have been caught doping with GH. The anabolic and metabolic effects make GH and IGF-1 attractive performance-enhancing drugs. The known changes in body composition coupled with effects on intermediate metabolism provide a theoretical basis for their misuse. Only recently has the scientific evidence started to catch up with the athletes' perception that these hormones are enhancing performance.

Acknowledgements

R.I.G.H. is the principal investigator of the GH-2004 project, which has developed a test for GH misuse. A.R.N. is a research fellow of the GH-2004 project. The GH-2004 study has received funding from WADA, the US Anti-Doping Agency, and the Partnership for Clean Competition.

References

1 Holt R, Sönksen P: Growth hormone, IGF-I and insulin and their abuse in sport. Br J Pharmacol 2008; 154:542–546.
2 Saugy M, Robinson N, Mangin P: Human growth hormone doping in sport. Br J Sports Med 2006l;40(suppl 1):135–139.
3 McHugh C, Park R, Sönksen P, Holt R: Challenges in detecting the abuse of growth hormone in sport. Clin Chem 2005;51:1587–1593.
4 Sonksen P: Insulin, growth hormone and sport. J Endocrinol 2001;170:13–25.
5 Erotokritou-Mulligan I, Guha N, Stow M, Bassett E, Bartlett C, Cowan D, et al: The development of decision limits for the implementation of the GH-2000 detection methodology using current commercial insulin-like growth factor and amino-terminal propeptide of type III collagen assays. Growth Horm IGF Res 2012;22:53–58.
6 Duchaine D: Underground Steroid Handbook II. Venice, HLR Technical Books, 1989.
7 Mitchell G: Report to the Commissioner of Baseball of an Independent Investigation into the Illegal use of Steroids and Other Performance Enhancing Substances by Players in Major League Baseball. Office of the Commissioner of Baseball, 2007, http://files.mlb.com/mitchrpt.pdf.
8 Fainaru-Wada M, Williams L: Game of Shadows. New York, Gotham Books, 2007.
9 Kelso P: UK Anti-Doping's first positive test for human growth hormone a boost for London 2012. Daily Telegraph, Feb 22, 2010.
10 Erotokritou-Mulligan E, Holt R, Sonksen P: Growth hormone doping: a review. J Sports Med 2011;2:99–111.
11 Cassoni P, Papotti M, Ghè C, Catapano F, Sapino A, Graziani A, Deghenghi R, Reissmann T, Ghigo E, Mucciolo G: Identification, characterization, and biological activity of specific receptors for natural (ghrelin) and synthetic growth hormone secretagogues and analogs in human breast carcinomas and cell lines 1. J Clin Endocrinol Metab 2001;86:1738–1745.
12 Smith RG: Development of growth hormone secretagogues. Endocr Rev 2005;26:346–360.
13 Thevis M, Wilkens F, Geyer H, Schanzer W: Determination of therapeutics with growth-hormone secretagogue activity in human urine for doping control purposes. Rapid Commun Mass Spectrom 2006; 20:3393–3402.
14 Giustina A, Mazziotti G, Canalis E: Growth hormone, insulin-like growth factors, and the skeleton. Endocr Rev 2008;29:535–539.
15 Vijayakumar A, Novosyadlyy R, Wu Y, Yakar S, LeRoith D: Biological effects of growth hormone on carbohydrate and lipid metabolism. Growth Horm IGF Res 2010;20:1–7.
16 Takaya K, Ariyasu H, Kanamoto N, Iwakura H, Yoshimoto A, Harada M, Mori K, et al: Ghrelin strongly stimulates growth hormone release in humans. J Clin Endocrinol Metab 2000;85:4908–4911.
17 Daughaday W: Growth hormone axis overview – somatomedin hypothesis. Paediatr Nephrol 2000;14: 537–540.
18 Moller N, Jorgensen J: Effects of growth hormone on glucose, lipid, and protein metabolism in human subjects. Endocr Rev 2009;30:152–177.
19 Clemmons D: Metabolic actions of insulin-like growth factor-I in normal physiology and diabetes. Endocrinol Metab Clin North Am 2012;41:425–443.
20 Bratusch-Marrain P, Smith D, DeFronzo R: The effect of growth hormone on glucose metabolism and insulin secretion in man. J Clin Endocrinol Metab 1982;55:973–982.
21 Clemmons D: The relative roles of growth hormone and IGF-1 in controlling insulin sensitivity. J Clin Invest 2004;113:25–27.
22 Agha A, Monson J: Modulation of glucocorticoid metabolism by the growth hormone-IGF-I axis. Clin Endocrinol (Oxf) 2007;66:459–465.
23 Ohlsson C, Bengtsson B, Isaksson O, Adreasson T, et al: Growth hormone and bone. Endocr Rev 1998;19: 55–79.
24 Mohan S, Richman C, Guo R, Amaar Y, Donahue L, Wergedal J, Baylink D: Insulin-like growth factor regulates peak bone mineral density in mice by both growth hormone-dependent and -independent mechanisms. Endocrinology 2003;144:929–936.
25 Landin-Wilhelmsen K, Nilsson A, Bosaueus I, Bengtsson B: Growth hormone increases bone mineral content in postmenopausal osteoporosis: a randomized placebo-controlled trial. J Bone Miner Res 2003;18:393–405.
26 Weissberger A, Anastasiadis A, Sturgess I, Martin F, Smith M, Sönksen P: Recombinant human growth hormone treatment in elderly patients undergoing elective total hip replacement. Clin Endocrinol (Oxf) 2003;58:99–107.
27 Gotherstrom G, Bengtsson BA, Bosaeus I, Johannsson G, Svensson J: A 10-year prospective study of the metabolic effects of growth hormone replacement in adults. J Clin Endocrinol Metab 2007;92:1442–1445.
28 Götherström G, Bengtsson BA, Bosaeus I, Johannsson G, Svensson J: Ten-year GH replacement increases bone mineral density in hypopituitary patients with adult onset GH deficiency. Eur J Endocrinol 2007;156:55–64.

29 Gibney J, Healy M, Sönksen P: The growth hormone/insulin-like growth factor-I axis in exercise and sport. Endocr Rev 2008;228:603–624.
30 Frystyk J: Exercise and the growth hormone-insulin-like growth factor axis. Med Sci Sports Exerc 2010; 42:58–66.
31 Pasarica M, Zachwieja J, DeJonge L, Redman S, et al: Effect of growth hormone on body composition and visceral adiposity in middle-aged men with visceral obesity. J Clin Endocrinol Metab 2007;92:4265–4270.
32 Sattler F, Casteneda-Sceppa C, Binder E, Schroeder T, Wang Y, et al: Testosterone and growth hormone improve body composition and muscle performance in older men. J Clin Endocrinol Metab 2009;94: 1991–2001.
33 Liu H, Bravata D, Olkin L, Friedlander A, Liu V, Roberts B, et al: Systematic review: the effects of growth hormone on athletic performance. Ann Intern Med 2008;148:747–758.
34 Thompson JL, Butterfield GE, Gylfadottir UK, Yesavage J, Marcus R, Hintz RL, Pearman A, Hoffman AR: Effects of growth hormone, insulin-like growth factor I and diet and exercise on body composition of obese postmenopausal women. J Clin Endocrinol Metab 1998;83:1477–1484.
35 Mauras N, O'Brien KO, Welch S, Rini A, Helgeson K, Vieira NE, Yergey AL: Insulin-like growth factor I and growth hormone (GH) treatment in GH-deficient humans: differential effects on protein, glucose, lipid, and calcium metabolism. J Clin Endocrinol Metab 2000;85:1686–1694.
36 Guha N, Nevitt P, Francis M, Woodland J, Böhning D, Sönksen P, Holt RI: The effects of recombinant human insulin-like growth factor-I/insulin-like growth factor binding protein-3 administration on body composition and physical fitness in recreational athletes. J Clin Endocrinol Metab 2015;100:3126–3131.
37 Widdowson W, Gibney J: The effect of growth hormone replacement on exercise capacity in patients with GH deficiency: a metaanalysis. J Clin Endocrinol Metab 2008;93:4413–4417.
38 Graham MR, Baker JS, Evans P, Kicman A, Cowan D, Hullin D, et al: Physical effects of short-term recombinant human growth hormone administration in abstinent steroid dependency. Horm Res 2008;69: 343–354.
39 Meinhardt U, Nelson AE, Hansen JL, Birzniece V, Clifford D, Leung KC, et al: The effects of growth hormone on body composition and physical performance in recreational athletes: a randomized trial. Ann Intern Med 2010;152:568–577.
40 Powrie J, Weissberger A, Sönksen P: Growth hormone replacement therapy for growth hormone-deficient adults. Drugs 1995;49:656–663.
41 Jenkins PJ, Mukherjee A, Shalet SM: Does growth hormone cause cancer? Clin Endocrinol (Oxf) 2006; 64:115–121.
42 Brown P, Gajdusek DC, Gibbs CJ Jr, Asher DM: Potential epidemic of Creutzfeldt-Jakob disease from human growth hormone therapy. N Engl J Med 1985;313:728–731.
43 Boonen S, Rosen C, Bouillon R, Sommer A, McKay M, Rosen D, Adams S, et al: Musculoskeletal effects of rhIGF-I/IGF binding protein-3 complex in osteoporotic patients with proximal femoral fracture: a double-blind, placebo-controlled pilot study. J Clin Endocrinol Metab 2002;87:1593–1599.

Dr. Adam R. Nicholls
The Institute for Developmental Sciences (MP887), Southampton General Hospital
Tremona Road
Southampton SO16 6YD (UK)
E-Mail adam.nicholls@uhs.nhs.uk

Use of Performance-Enhancing Endocrine Drugs (Doping) in Competitive and Recreational Sports Activity

Lanfranco F, Strasburger CJ (eds): Sports Endocrinology.
Front Horm Res. Basel, Karger, 2016, vol 47, pp 115–127 (DOI: 10.1159/000445174)

Erythropoietin

Wolfgang Jelkmann

Institute of Physiology, University of Lübeck, Lübeck, Germany

Abstract

Total hemoglobin (Hb) mass is an important determinant of aerobic power. The glycoprotein erythropoietin (Epo) promotes the production of red blood cells (RBCs). The present article reviews the regulation of erythropoiesis and ways of its manipulation. The various Epos, e.g. recombinant human (rh)Epo and (epoetin), and their long-acting analogues can be misused by cheating athletes, but the drugs are detectable by chemical tests, because their glycan isoform structures differ from those of endogenous Epo. Still, anti-doping control has become more difficult, since additional erythropoiesis-stimulating agents have become available (Epo mimetics, activin inhibitors, and small-molecule chemical drugs activating *EPO* expression). A major problem is created by hypoxia-inducible factor (HIF) stabilizers (e.g. α-ketoglutarate competitors and Co^{2+} salt) which activate HIFs and thus increase *EPO* expression. Direct *EPO* transfer is theoretically also possible but medically little advanced. To overcome weaknesses of direct testing of biological fluids, the World Anti-Doping Agency has implemented the Athlete Biological Passport for continuous monitoring of RBC parameters of athletes. Blood doping is assumed when distinct parameters (blood Hb concentration and reticulocytes) change in a nonphysiological way.

Red blood cells (RBCs) circulate for 100–120 days in the human organism. Then, they are engulfed by macrophages. About 1% of the 25×10^{12} erythrocytes of an adult are removed every day. They are replaced by reticulocytes originating from the red bone marrow. Hence, RBC numbers, blood hemoglobin (Hb) concentration and O_2 capacity are constant in health. Erythropoiesis requires the presence of the glycoprotein erythropoietin (Epo). Under normal conditions, the concentration of this hormone is only $\sim 10^{-11}$ mol/l in blood plasma. However, this value can increase by to up to three orders of magnitude under hypoxic conditions.

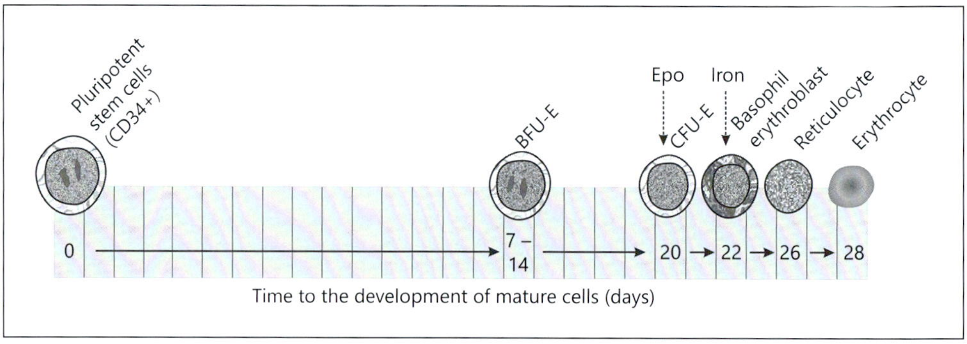

Fig. 1. Time frame of developmental steps between CD34+ hematopoietic stem cells and erythrocytes. Note that each developmental step is associated with cell division until the nucleus is extruded by the late normoblast (>20 cell divisions). Starting about 4 days after an increase in Epo levels, more reticulocytes enter the blood stream. In addition to Epo, iron is of major importance for effective erythropoiesis.

Because the aerobic capacity of athletes correlates with total Hb mass (Hb_{mass}), some athletes apply forbidden substances and techniques to increase their Hb concentration [1]. This article reviews the regulation of erythropoiesis and describes ways of its manipulation.

Structure and Function of Erythropoietin

Epo is a 30.4-kDa glycoprotein of 165 amino acids, three tetra-antennary N-linked glycans (at Asn^{24}, Asn^{38}, and Asn^{83}) and one small O-linked glycan (at Ser^{126}). The N-glycans are critical for the secretion, molecular stability, receptor binding, and in vivo bioactivity of Epo. Both endogenous Epo and recombinant human (rh)Epo exhibit several glycosylation isoforms which can be detected by electrophoresis or isoelectric focusing (IEF) followed by immunoblotting.

As shown in figure 1, RBCs are the offspring of CD34+ hematopoietic stem cells, also called 'CFU-GEMMs' (colony-forming units generating granulocytes, erythrocytes, monocytes, and megakaryocytes). The human bone marrow hosts about 5×10^5 hematopoietic stem cells, and these give rise to about 2×10^{11} RBCs every day – amongst the many other myeloid blood cells. The 'BFU-Es' (burst-forming unit erythroids) are the earliest cells of the erythrocytic compartment. The 'CFU-Es' (colony-forming unit erythroids), which follow the BFU-Es, express abundant Epo receptor (Epo-R) molecules. CFU-Es undergo apoptosis in the absence of Epo, whereas in the presence of Epo, CFU-Es and their progeny divide several times generating 8–64 erythroblasts within 7–8 days. Once the level of 'orthochromatic erythroblasts' (synonymous with 'normoblasts') is reached, the cells do not divide any more but extrude their nuclei and become reticulocytes. Within 1–2 days after their release into the

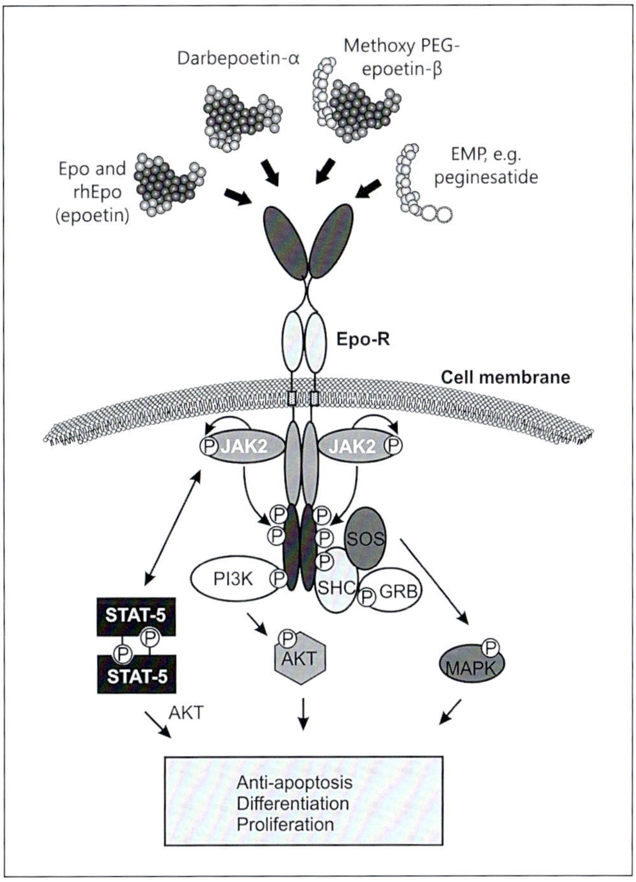

Fig. 2. Scheme of Epo receptor signaling. Endogenous Epo, its recombinant analogues, and EMPs can bind to the homodimeric Epo-R. Epo-R then recruits JAK2 that catalyzes Epo-R/JAK2 transphosphorylation to activate STAT-5, PI3K/AKT, and SHC/MAPK pathways. STAT-5 induces the expression of anti-apoptotic proteins (for example Bcl-x_L). PI3K and MAPK prevent pro-apoptotic proteins (Bax and Bad) from activating caspases. MAPK activates genes promoting cell proliferation (reproduced with permission [31]).

circulation, reticulocytes mature to erythrocytes, which have no organelles and are smaller.

As shown in figure 2, the human Epo-R, a membrane-spanning ~59-kDa glycoprotein (484-amino-acid residues and 1 N-glycan), is a member of the cytokine receptor superfamily I and acts as homodimer [2]. Epo binding causes the intracellular activation of Epo-R-associated Janus kinase 2 (JAK2). In turn, JAK2, Epo-R, and other cytosolic proteins are tyrosyl-phosphorylated by tyrosine. The phosphorylated Epo-R provides docking sites for proteins containing SRC homology 2 (SH2) domains. Epo-R signaling involves signal transducer and activator of transcription 5 (STAT-5), phosphatidylinositol 3-kinase (PI3K)/AKT, and SHC (SH2 adaptor protein C)/mitogen-activated protein kinase (MAPK).

The action of Epo is terminated when the Epo/Epo-R-complex is internalized following Epo-R dephosphorylation by the tyrosine phosphatase SHP-1 (Src homology phosphatase-1). Epo-R-mediated Epo uptake by its target cells is a major mechanism of the removal of Epo from the circulation. Reticulocytes and mature erythrocytes lack Epo-R.

Role of Iron

Healthy humans have about 3–4 g of iron, with women having less than men. Most of the iron – about 2.5 g – is incorporated in the heme structures of the Hb. The daily loss of 2 mg/day in healthy women (with regular menstrual bleeding) and of 1 mg/day in men is counterbalanced by absorption of dietary iron (Fe^{2+}). In the blood plasma, the then oxidized iron (Fe^{3+}) is carried by the hepatic 678-amino-acid glycoprotein transferrin (79.5 kDa), which delivers it to cells via specific transferrin receptors (TfRs). The serum transferrin Fe^{3+} saturation and the levels of soluble TfR and ferritin in serum provide information on the rate of erythropoiesis and the body iron status. Soluble TfR is elevated under conditions of increased erythropoiesis. Serum ferritin of 12 µg/l or less is generally indicative of iron deficiency. However, because ferritin is an acute-phase protein, its concentration may be elevated due to inflammation. Thus, a low mean Hb content in reticulocytes is the most reliable indicator of iron deficiency.

Iron homeostasis is under the control of the hormone hepcidin, a peptide of 25-amino-acid residues. It binds to the cell surface iron export protein ferroportin, thereby causing its internalization and proteolytic degradation. Hepcidin production increases primarily in conditions of iron overload, hypoxia, or inflammation. Recently, the glycoprotein erythroferrone with 326-amino-acid residues has been identified as another regulator of iron homeostasis [3]. Erythroferrone is produced by erythrocytic progenitors in response to Epo to increase iron absorption and mobilization of iron from stores. The administration of rhEpo causes hepcidin down-regulation within 24 h [4].

Sites and Control of Epo Production

Peritubular fibroblasts in the renal cortex are the main site of Epo synthesis. In addition, the liver, spleen, bone marrow, brain, and other organs can express Epo mRNA in small amounts. The concentration of circulating Epo increases exponentially with decreasing Hb concentration in uncomplicated anemia (absence of renal disease or inflammation). The critical parameter is the tissue oxygen tension (pO_2), which depends on the arterial pO_2, Hb concentration, and Hb-O_2 affinity (fig. 3). The rate of renal blood flow is less significant, here, because renal O_2 consumption decreases in proportion with blood flow.

The human Epo gene (*EPO*; on chromosome 7q22) is under the control of several transcription factors. The *EPO* promoter is inhibited by GATA-2 and by nuclear factor κB which reduce *EPO* expression in inflammatory diseases. Most important is the *EPO* enhancer, which possesses a hypoxia response element and is activated by hypoxia-inducible factors (HIFs). One HIF α-subunit and a HIF-1β subunit (each 100–120 kDa) can form heterodimers in the cell nuclei. There are at least three

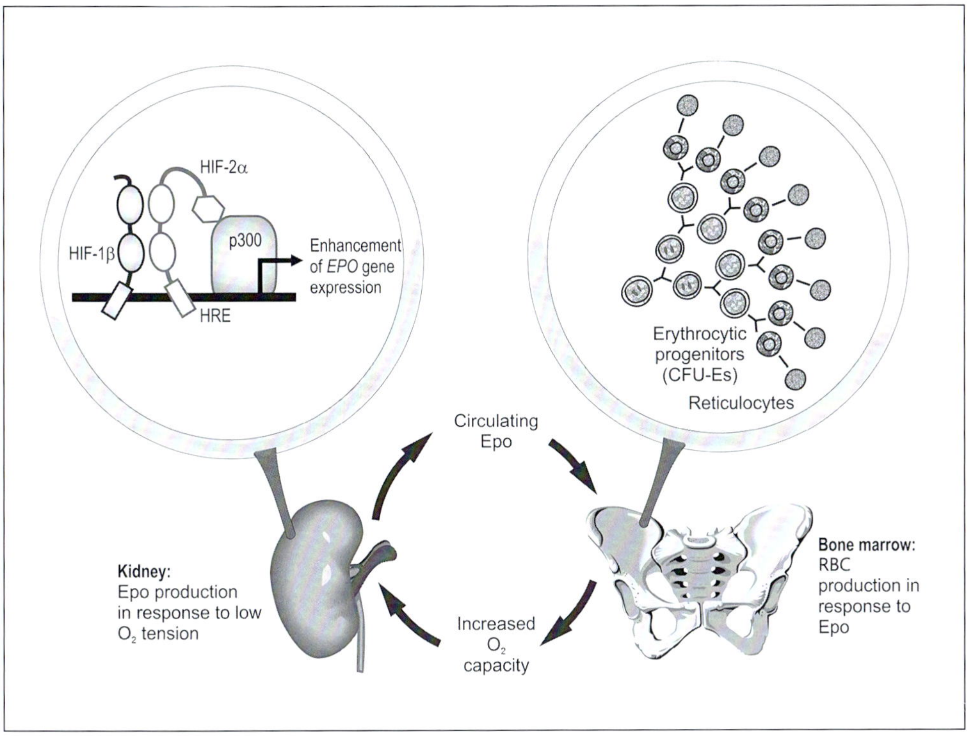

Fig. 3. Scheme of erythropoiesis. The kidneys are the main site of Epo production. The *EPO* enhancer is activated by the HIF-2α/HIF-1β complex. Supported by cofactors such as p300, the HIF complex binds to the hypoxia-response element (HRE) activating *EPO* expression. In the bone marrow, Epo promotes survival, proliferation, and differentiation of erythrocytic progenitors, particularly CFU-Es (reproduced with permission [31]).

different HIF-α isoforms. HIF-1 (-1α/-1β) plays major roles in metabolic processes, such as glucose metabolism, whereas HIF-2 (-2α/-1β) is more restricted to specific cell types, including the Epo-producing renal fibroblasts [5]. HIF-1α, HIF-2α, and HIF-1β are constantly translated. However, HIF-α subunits are usually missing under normoxic conditions, because they are O_2 labile. Their C-terminus contains two prolyl residues (e.g. Pro^{405} and Pro^{531} in HIF-2α) that are hydroxylated by specific prolyl-4-hydroxylase domain proteins (PHD-1, -2, and -3) in the presence of O_2. Prolyl-hydroxylated HIF-α undergoes immediate proteasomal degradation, as it is recognized by the von Hippel-Lindau tumor suppressor protein in association with an E3 ubiquitin ligase. Under hypoxic conditions, the HIF-α subunits translocate into the nucleus and dimerize with HIF-1β. The transcriptional activity of HIFs is further attenuated by O_2-dependent enzymatic hydroxylation of an asparaginyl residue (Asn^{847} in HIF-2α) by the so-called 'factor inhibiting HIF'. As a result of this hydroxylation, binding of the transcriptional coactivator p300-CBP (CREB-binding protein) to the HIF complexes is prevented (fig. 3). The HIF-α hydroxylases are Fe^{2+}-

containing dioxygenases that require α-ketoglutarate as cofactor. Competitors of α-ketoglutarate (HIF stabilizers) prevent HIF-α degradation and stimulate Epo production.

Epo concentrations increase exponentially with decreasing blood Hb concentrations in otherwise healthy subjects. Epo values may rise to 10,000 IU/l in severe anemia (normal value: ~6–32 IU/l). *EPO* expression is also stimulated when the arterial pO_2 decreases or when the O_2 affinity of the blood is abnormally high. The plasma Epo level increases during acclimatization to high altitude, with peak values 1–2 days after the ascent. Thereafter, erythropoiesis remains to be elevated although the Epo concentration is little increased at continued altitude residence. Training and/or residence at high altitude (or in artificially O_2-deprived chambers at sea level) have been applied to improve the aerobic power of athletes. However, the benefit derived from an enhanced O_2 capacity is eventually offset by the increase in blood viscosity, which can be extreme in chronic mountain sickness.

Effect of Physical Exercise on Erythropoiesis

The plasma Epo level is not usually affected by single bouts of strenuous exercise at sea level. It is plausible that there are no major effects of normoxic exercise on Epo production, since the O_2 sensor controlling Epo synthesis is not located in skeletal muscles or the heart but in the kidneys. Generally, there are no major differences in basal RBC count, hematocrit (Hct), blood Hb concentration, and mean corpuscular Hb concentration (MCHC) in athletes in comparison to nonathletes, but Hb_{mass} is increased in elite endurance athletes [1]. In contrast, sportsmen, particularly those practicing endurance sports, may present with relatively low Hb concentrations and Hct values. This 'sports anemia' is usually a pseudoanemia due to an enlarged plasma volume. If there is an increased rate of intravascular hemolysis caused by compression, the RBC lifespan will be reduced.

Misuse of Erythropoiesis-Stimulating Agents

Because Hb_{mass} correlates with aerobic capacity, some athletes seek to increase erythropoiesis by pharmacological means (table 1). Treatment with rhEpo or other erythropoiesis-stimulating agents (ESAs) may enhance performance by raising Hb concentration. Studies show that following the administration of low-dose rhEpo to healthy volunteers, maximal O_2 uptake (O_{2max}) is increased by 6–12% when Hct is raised to approximately 0.50. In addition, the time to exhaustion (in the laboratory) is increased by up to 50% at a given level of O_{2max} [6]. When rhEpo administration is discontinued, O_{2max} remains elevated for at least 3 weeks. ESAs are particularly effective in combination with supplemental iron.

Table 1. Erythropoiesis-stimulating substances and techniques prohibited in sports

Compound/technique	Manufacturing procedure	Marketing status
Recombinant products		
Epoetins (e.g. α or β)	*EPO*-transfected mammalian cells (mostly CHO)	Marketed globally
Methoxy PEG-epoetin-β	*EPO*-transfected CHO cells, posttranslational modification	Marketed in EU and Asia
Darbepoetin-α	Mutated *EPO*-transfected CHO cells, hyperglycosylated	Marketed globally
SEP	Chemical synthesis, polymer coupled	In preclinical trials
Epo fusion proteins (Epo-Epo, Epo-Fc, Epo-β-hCG)	Recombinant DNA technology	In clinical trials
Epo mimetics		
Peptidic	Chemical synthesis or recombinant	In clinical trials
Nonpeptidic	Chemical synthesis	In preclinical trials
Activin inhibitors (sotatercept)	Recombinant DNA technology	In clinical trials
Epo gene activators		
GATA antagonists	Chemical synthesis	In preclinical trials
HIF stabilizers	Small orally active molecules, chemical synthesis or natural (e.g. Co^{2+})	In clinical trials
EPO transfer	Ex vivo gene transfer	In clinical trials
	In vivo gene transfer	In preclinical trials

CHO = Chinese hamster ovary; SEP = synthetic erythropoiesis protein.

The use of ESAs for doping purposes is forbidden, and their presence can be proven by chemical tests [7]. However, there are several low-cost small-molecule substances capable of stimulating erythropoiesis (table 1). Of particular concern are substances that induce *EPO* expression, such as cobalt(II) ions (Co^{2+}). This action of cobalt is fully separate from that of cobalamin (vitamin B_{12}). Co^{2+} stabilizes HIF-α, thereby increasing *EPO* expression [8].

Recombinant Erythropoiesis-Stimulating Agents

Recombinant ESAs have been developed for clinical use, i.e. for the treatment of anemias associated with chronic kidney disease or cancer treated with myelosuppressive chemotherapy. Several products are available. 'Epoetin' is the international nonproprietary drug name (INN) for eukaryotic cell-derived rhEpo, whose amino acid sequence is identical with that of endogenous human Epo. Differences in the amino acid residue chain are indicated by a random prefix (e.g. *darb*epoetin). Differences in production processes and glycosylation patterns may be indicated by Greek letters (e.g. α or β). However, the Greek lettering has not been standardized globally, as identical epoetins may differ in INN while different epoetins can have the same INN.

Following intravenous administration, epoetins are eliminated at a first-order kinetic rate following the rapid distribution (volume of distribution 0.03–0.09 liters/kg body weight). Following subcutaneous administration, peak plasma concentrations of rhEpo are achieved after 12–18 h, with bioavailability amounting to about 30%. There are recombinant ESAs with prolonged survival in the circulation, which provides clinical benefits. Darbepoetin-α is a hyperglycosylated analogue (37.1 kDa), which contains two additional N-glycans in association with an exchange of 5 amino acids. Compared with the terminal half-life of intravenously administered epoetin (6–9 h), the half-life of darbepoetin-α is 3- to 4-fold longer (25 h). Another long-acting ESA is methoxy polyethylene glycol (PEG)-epoetin-β. The half-life of methoxy PEG-epoetin-β (60 kDa) amounts to 130–140 h on intravenous injection. The prolonged in vivo survival of darbepoetin-α and methoxy PEG-epoetin-β is in part due to a reduced Epo-R binding affinity.

Recombinant ESAs can be demonstrated by IEF and immunoblotting of urine samples [7]. Endogenous Epo presents with more acidic isoforms than the epoetins. Darbepoetin-α migrates even more in the acidic range than endogenous Epo. IEF of methoxy PEG-epoetin-β yields bands in the less acidic area when compared to endogenous Epo. Of note, once the blood Hb concentration has been raised artificially (by RBC transfusion or ESA administration), only very low ESA doses are needed to maintain the elevated Hb concentration. In this situation, the window of detection of regular epoetin in urine is only 12–18 h [9]. Clearly, use of darbepoetin-α or methoxy PEG-epoetin-β is associated with a prolonged window of their detection, which makes these ESAs less eligible for blood doping. Methoxy PEG-epoetin-β is also detectable by IEF of blood serum [10].

Erythropoietin-Mimetic Peptides

Epo-mimetic peptides (EMPs) are synthetic cyclic peptides of about 20 amino acids that signal through Epo-R (fig. 2) but show no sequence homology to Epo. The clinically most advanced product was peginesatide, a pegylated homodimer of two EMPs (each ~2 kDa, total mass 45 kDa). The product was initially approved in the USA for treatment of anemic patients with chronic renal failure but subsequently recalled after the occurrence of lethal acute hypersensitivity reactions in several patients. It is questionable whether other EMPs will become available for human use in the near future [11].

Activin Inhibitors

Sotatercept (ACE-011) is a novel recombinant erythropoietic protein. It is composed of the extracellular part of the activin type II receptor and the Fc domain of human IgG1. In a clinical phase I study, single intravenous injections of sotatercept proved to increase blood Hb levels, RBC numbers, and Hct [12]. However, the mechanisms underlying the effect of sotatercept or analogous compounds on erythropoiesis are still poorly understood. Cellular or soluble factors in the bone marrow microenvironment could be involved [11, 13].

GATA Antagonists

EPO expression can be stimulated by GATA antagonists. These are organic small-molecule compounds that prevent GATA-2 from suppressing the *EPO* promoter. For example, the diazepane derivative K-7174 acts this way. Its follow-on product K-11706 was shown to be effective in increasing physical performance of mice [14]. However, human studies have not been reported with GATA antagonists.

Hypoxia-Inducible Factor Stabilizers

α-Ketoglutarate competitors and Fe^{2+} chelators inhibit the degradation of HIF-α proteins, because α-ketoglutarate and Fe^{2+} are required for HIF-α prolyl- and asparaginyl-hydroxylation [15]. Such HIF-stabilizing substances promote the transcription of HIF-dependent genes even under normoxic conditions. Fe^{2+} chelators are not appropriate to increase Hb levels, as Fe^{2+} is required for heme synthesis. In contrast, HIF-stabilizing α-ketoglutarate competitors stimulate erythropoiesis by increasing *EPO* expression in the kidneys and at extrarenal sites. Effects of one of the compounds (FG-2216) has been demonstrated in a phase I clinical trial [16]. Other HIF stabilizers are under development [11]. Advantages of the HIF stabilizers (compared to recombinant proteins) include the oral route of administration. However, HIFs can activate >1,000 genes apart from *EPO*, including genes for proteins that are involved in tumor growth, such as vascular endothelial growth factor [17]. On the other hand, some of the HIF-activated genes encode proteins (e.g. for glycolytic enzymes, glucose transporters, and angiogenic peptides) which may increase physical performance independent from the stimulation of erythropoiesis (fig. 4).

The action of cobalt is of particular interest here. Co^{2+} binds to HIF-α, thereby preventing the interaction with the von Hippel-Lindau tumor suppressor protein and the degradation of HIF-α [8]. Intake of cobalt salt is probably the simplest means to stimulate HIF-dependent *EPO* expression. Per definition, 5 μmol Co^{2+} elicits the same erythropoiesis-stimulating activity as 1 IU Epo. Cobalt salt is inexpensive and readily available. In earlier days, it was administered as tablets (mostly cobalt chloride; at daily doses of up to 300 mg) for anemia treatment [18]. Typical adverse effects associated with chronic Co^{2+} intake include nausea, vomiting, heart failure, hypothyroidism, and goiter. Doses of (at least) 10–25 mg cobalt chloride are required to stimulate Epo production. Cobalt doping also has its role in sports involving animals. Of note, one has to differentiate between the potential of Co^{2+} to stabilize HIF-α and the role of cobalt as part of cobalamin (vitamin B_{12}) [8]. Cobalamin supplementation has no proven beneficial effect on performance in the absence of a nutritional cobalamin deficit.

There has been public suspicion that inhalation of xenon could stimulate Epo production by activating HIF. In fact, in 2014, the World Anti-Doping Agency (WADA)

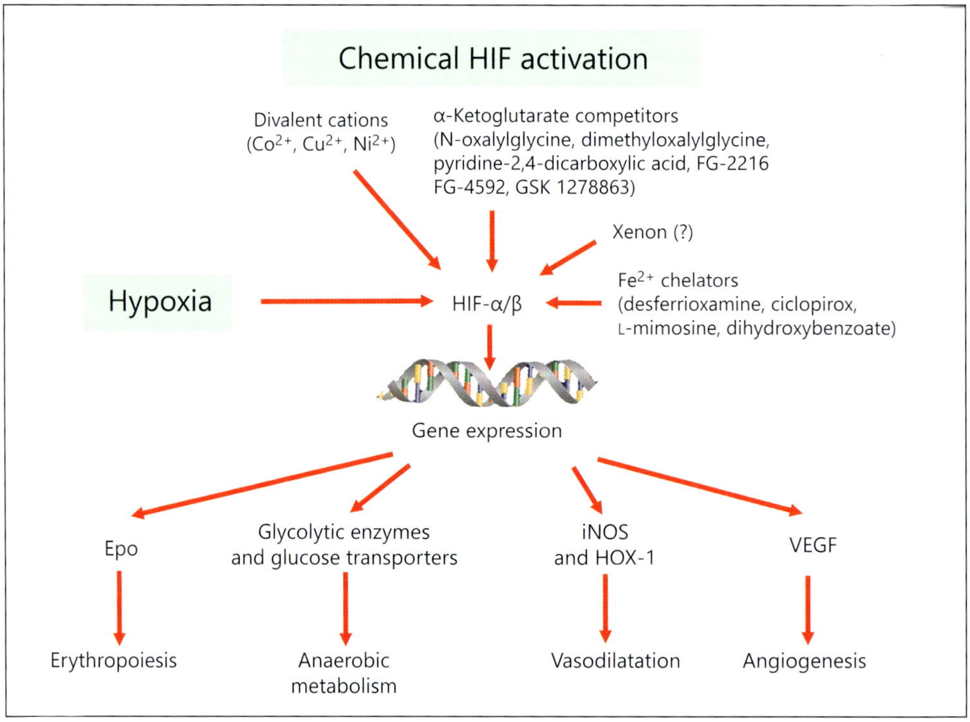

Fig. 4. Overview of compounds that may stimulate HIF-dependent gene expression and functional consequences. HOX-1 = Heme oxygenase-1; iNOS = inducible nitric oxide synthase; VEGF = vascular endothelial growth factor.

List Committee approved the option to modify section S.2. of the 'Prohibited List', where xenon and argon have now been specifically identified as HIF activators. However, there is no evidence from human studies indicating xenon is indeed effective in stimulating erythropoiesis [19].

EPO Gene Transfer

In vivo allogeneic *EPO* transfer can cause immune reactions. Furthermore, it may be detected when applied by athletes. Unusual Epo glycosylation forms were detected following adeno-associated virus-mediated allogeneic *EPO* transfer into skeletal muscle of cynomolgus macaques [20]. Furthermore, anti-doping research has provided techniques to specifically amplify intron-less DNA sequences allowing the detection of small amounts of transgenic DNA in blood [21, 22].

Ex vivo *EPO* transfer is performed by use of transfected autologous or allogeneic cells that are transferred from in vitro cultures into the individual. The autologous ex vivo approach has been investigated in clinical trials [23]. Thereby, individual dermal core samples (biopumps) were incubated in vitro with *EPO* cDNA inserted into a vector containing the cytomegalovirus promoter and the simian virus-40 polyA site.

However, the method has made little progress and not stepped beyond the clinical trial phase after many years of study.

Taken together, due to technical difficulties, gene doping with *EPO* is probably not applied in sports so far [24].

Effects of Erythropoietin on Red Blood Cell Parameters

Pharmacological stimulation of erythropoiesis may cause iron-deficient erythropoiesis, which, in the presence of adequate iron stores, is termed 'functional iron deficiency' [25]. This is indicated by the production of erythrocytes with low Hb content and concentration (hypochromic cells). Modern blood analyzers enable to measure mean corpuscular volume of reticulocytes (in fl) and MCHC (in g/l), and to calculate the mean Hb content of reticulocytes (in pg, normal range: 28.5–34.5 pg). Increases in the percentage of hypochromic RBCs with a Hb concentration <280 g/l (normal range: 0–4.8%) and reticulocytes presenting with a mean Hb content of reticulocytes <28 pg indicate functional iron deficiency more accurately than serum iron transferrin saturation or ferritin concentrations [25].

The efficacy of ESA administration is augmented by intravenous iron administration. As shown in the early days of rhEpo research, Hb concentrations, RBC numbers, Hct, hypochromic macrocyte counts, and the percentage of reticulocytes (Ret%) increase significantly when athletes receive rhEpo at common doses of 30 U kg^{-1} body weight s.c. every other day for 30–45 days, along with twice weekly iron (62 mg i.v.) and oral vitamins [26]. The validity of the use of reticulocyte counts for anti-doping purposes and also for evaluating health status and iron metabolism of sportsmen has been established.

Irrespective of the misuse of ESAs, the immature reticulocyte fraction shows a tendency to be increased in athletes [27] owing to continuous bone marrow stimulation linked to increased hemolysis in some sport disciplines. In addition, low-dose treatment with rhEpo (about 15 IU kg^{-1} three times a week) did not increase Ret% above normal in subjects with elevated Hb concentrations due to previously high doses of rhEpo [9]. Ret% usually decrease to very low values on cessation of ESA administration due to the feedback control of Epo production (fig. 3; table 2).

Biological Passport of the World Anti-Doping Agency

Traditional anti-doping analyses are based on the demonstration of a substance in biological fluids (adverse analytical finding). This approach has several limitations regarding blood doping. Autologous RBC transfusion is not directly detectable, there is a plethora of different ESAs, the time frame for their detection is limited, they can be used at low dose and in combination, and there may be urine manipulation. Therefore, WADA has implemented the 'Athlete Biological Passport' (ABP) in 2009. The

Table 2. Indicators of ESA doping and blood transfusions (according to Sottas et al. [32])

Indicator	ESA doping		Blood transfusions	
	stimulation	maintenance	withdrawal	re-infusion
Blood Hb	↑	↑	↓	↑
Hct	↑	↑	↓	↑
Erythrocyte counts	↑	↑	↓	↑
Ret%	↑	↓	↑	↓
OFFS	↔	↑	↓	↑

↑ = Increase; ↓ = decrease; ↔ = no change.

ABP is based on individual and longitudinal monitoring of blood and urine markers. Blood doping is suspected when these parameters change in a nonphysiological way (table 2). The ABP Operating Guidelines include annexes which compile mandatory protocols that must be followed by the Anti-Doping Organizations using the ABP.

The following markers have been included in the hematological ABP module: Hct, Hb concentration, RBC count, Ret%, reticulocyte count, mean corpuscular volume, Hb count, MCHC, and OFF-hr score (OFFS). The OFFS is an index of stimulation derived from the formula: Hb concentration (g/l) – 60 × $\sqrt{\text{Ret\%}}$; its normal range amounts to 85–95, with an upper normal value <113.5 [28]. Abnormal Hb concentrations and OFFS patterns fulfill the conditions to potentially sanction an athlete. Indeed, as Hb concentrations show normally little intra-individual variation, larger deviations are suspicious for doping. The OFFS can expose cheating athletes, because it increases in a typical way on cessation of effective ESA use [29, 30].

References

1 Jelkmann W, Lundby C: Blood doping and its detection. Blood 2011;118:2395–2240.

2 Elliott S, Sinclair A: The effect of erythropoietin on normal and neoplastic cells. Biologics 2012;6:163–189.

3 Kautz L, Jung G, Nemeth E, Ganz T: Erythroferrone contributes to recovery from anemia of inflammation. Blood 2014;124:2569–2574.

4 Robach P, Recalcati S, Girelli D, Campostrini N, Kempf T, Wollert KC, Corbella M, Santambrogio P, Perbellini L, Brasse-Lagnel C, Christensen B, Moutereau S, Lundby C, Cairo G: Serum hepcidin levels and muscle iron proteins in humans injected with low- or high-dose erythropoietin. Eur J Haematol 2013;91:74–84.

5 Haase VH: Regulation of erythropoiesis by hypoxia-inducible factors. Blood Rev 2013;27:41–53.

6 Thomsen JJ, Rentsch RL, Robach P, Calbet JA, Boushel R, Rasmussen P, Juel C, Lundby C: Prolonged administration of recombinant human erythropoietin increases submaximal performance more than maximal aerobic capacity. Eur J Appl Physiol 2007;101:481–486.

7 Reichel C, Gmeiner G: Erythropoietin and analogs. Handb Exp Pharmacol 2010;195:251–294.

8 Jelkmann W: The disparate roles of cobalt in erythropoiesis, and doping relevance. Open J Hematol 2012, pp 3–6.

9 Ashenden M, Varlet-Marie E, Lasne F, Audran M: The effects of microdose recombinant human erythropoietin regimens in athletes. Haematologica 2006;91:1143–1144.

10 Lasne F, Martin L, Martin J, de Ceaurriz J: Isoelectric profiles of human erythropoietin are different in serum and urine. Int J Biol Macromol 2007;41:354–357.

11 Jelkmann W: The ESA scenario gets complex: from biosimilar epoetins to activin traps. Nephrol Dial Transplant 2015;30:553–559.
12 Ruckle J, Jacobs M, Kramer W, Pearsall AE, Kumar R, Underwood KW, Seehra J, Yang Y, Condon CH, Sherman ML: Single-dose, randomized, double-blind, placebo-controlled study of ACE-011 (ActRIIA-IgG1) in postmenopausal women. J Bone Miner Res 2009;24: 744–752.
13 Iancu-Rubin C, Mosoyan G, Wang J, Kraus T, Sung V, Hoffman R: Stromal cell-mediated inhibition of erythropoiesis can be attenuated by Sotatercept (ACE-011), an activin receptor type II ligand trap. Exp Hematol 2013;41:155–166.
14 Imagawa S, Matsumoto K, Horie M, Ohkoshi N, Nagasawa T, Doi T, Suzuki N, Yamamoto M: Does K-11706 enhance performance and why? Sports Med 2007;28:928–933.
15 Beuck S, Schänzer W, Thevis M: Hypoxia-inducible factor stabilizers and other small-molecule erythropoiesis-stimulating agents in current and preventive doping analysis. Drug Test Anal 2012;4:830–845.
16 Bernhardt WM, Wiesener MS, Scigalla P, Chou J, Schmieder RE, Gunzler V, Eckardt KU: Inhibition of prolyl hydroxylases increases erythropoietin production in ESRD. J Am Soc Nephrol 2010;21:2151–2156.
17 Ratcliffe PJ: Oxygen sensing and hypoxia signalling pathways in animals: the implications of physiology for cancer. J Physiol 2013;591:2027–2042.
18 Ebert B, Jelkmann W: Intolerability of cobalt salt as erythropoietic agent. Drug Test Anal 2014;6:185–189.
19 Jelkmann W: Xenon misuse in sports – increase of hypoxia-inducible factors and erythropoietin, or nothing but 'hot air'? Dtsch Z Sportmed 2014;65: 267–271.
20 Lasne F, Martin L, de Ceaurriz J, Larcher T, Moullier P, Chenuaud P: 'Genetic doping' with erythropoietin cDNA in primate muscle is detectable. Mol Ther 2004;10:409–410.
21 Beiter T, Zimmermann M, Fragasso A, Hudemann J, Niess AM, Bitzer M, Lauer UM, Simon P: Direct and long-term detection of gene doping in conventional blood samples. Gene Ther 2010;18:225–231.
22 Baoutina A, Coldham T, Bains GS, Emslie KR: Gene doping detection: evaluation of approach for direct detection of gene transfer using erythropoietin as a model system. Gene Ther 2010;17:1022–1032.
23 Lippin Y, Dranitzki-Elhalel M, Brill-Almon E, Mei-Zahav C, Mizrachi S, Liberman Y, Iaina A, Kaplan E, Podjarny E, Zeira E, Harati M, Casadevall N, Shani N, Galun E: Human erythropoietin gene therapy for patients with chronic renal failure. Blood 2005;106: 2280–2286.
24 Jelkmann W: Erythropoietin gene doping: facts and fictions. Sportwissenschaft 2012;42:280–285.
25 Schaefer RM, Schaefer L: Hypochromic red blood cells and reticulocytes. Kidney Int 1999;55:S44–S48.
26 Casoni I, Ricci G, Ballarin E, Borsetto C, Grazzi G, Guglielmini C, Manfredini F, Mazzoni G, Patracchini M, De Paoli Vitali E, Rigolin F, Bartalotta S, Franzè GP, Masotti M, Conconi F: Hematological indices of erythropoietin administration in athletes. Int J Sports Med 1993;14:307–311.
27 Banfi G, Del Fabbro M: Behaviour of reticulocyte counts and immature reticulocyte fraction during a competitive season in elite athletes of four different sports. Int J Lab Hematol 2007;29:127–131.
28 Saugy M, Lundby C, Robinson N: Monitoring of biological markers indicative of doping: the athlete biological passport. Br J Sports Med 2014;48:827–832.
29 Gore CJ, Parisotto R, Ashenden MJ, Stray-Gundersen J, Sharpe K, Hopkins W, Emslie KR, Howe C, Trout GJ, Kazlauskas R, Hahn AG: Second-generation blood tests to detect erythropoietin abuse by athletes. Haematologica 2003;88:333–344.
30 Parisotto R, Gore CJ, Hahn AG, Ashenden MJ, Olds TS, Martin DT, Pyne DB, Gawthorn K, Brugnara C: Reticulocyte parameters as potential discriminators of recombinant human erythropoietin abuse in elite athletes. Int J Sports Med 2000;21:471–479.
31 Jelkmann W: Physiology and pharmacology of erythropoietin. Transfus Med Hemother 2013;40: 302–309.
32 Sottas PE, Robinson N, Saugy M, Niggli O: A forensic approach to the interpretation of blood doping markers. Law Prob Risk 2008;7:191–210.

Wolfgang Jelkmann, MD
Institute of Physiology, University of Lübeck
Ratzeburger Allee 160
DE–23562 Lübeck (Germany)
E-Mail jelkmann@physio.uni-luebeck.de

Lanfranco F, Strasburger CJ (eds): Sports Endocrinology.
Front Horm Res. Basel, Karger, 2016, vol 47, pp 128–152 (DOI: 10.1159/000445176)

Ergogenic Aids and Supplements

Marisa Porrini · Cristian Del Bo'

Division of Human Nutrition, Department of Food, Environmental and Nutritional Sciences, Università degli Studi di Milano, Milan, Italy

Abstract

Great interest is currently shown for the contribution of nutrition to optimize training and athletic performance, and a considerable debate exists about the potential ergogenic value of several dietary supplements. However, most of the products used by athletes do not provide sufficient scientific evidence regarding their efficacy in enhancing physical performance as well as their specificity of action and safety. For this reason, sport nutrition professionals need skills in evaluating the scientific value of papers and advertisements on ergogenic aids and supplements in order to support athletes in their choice. In the present chapter, the efficacy of some of the most popular supplements used by athletes and sport practitioners will be discussed. Particular attention will be devoted to amino acids and derivatives, caffeine and caffeinated energy drinks, and some antioxidants.

An ergogenic aid is any training method, mechanical device, nutritional practice, pharmacological approach, or psychological technique that can improve exercise performance capacity and/or enhance training adaptations. This includes aids that may help prepare an individual to exercise, improve the efficiency of exercise, and/or enhance recovery from exercise [1].

Nowadays, great interest is shown for the contribution of nutrition to optimize training and athletic performance, and a considerable debate exists about the ergogenic value of various dietary supplements.

The use of dietary supplements is widespread, but individuals engaged in sport and physical activity represent a substantial portion of the population purchasing these products [2–4]. Dietary supplements can play an important role in helping athletes to

Table 1. Intake (%) of ergogenic substances and supplements in a group of individuals (n = 451) attending gyms (adapted from Leone and Pesce [8])

Substance	Total	Female	Male
Vitamins	53.4	53.1	54.6
Weight loss supplements	9.5	10.5	7.4
Proteins and amino-acid derivatives	12.4	7.8	19.6
Diuretics	4.0	4.7	3.0
Stimulants	17.8	20.7	13.5
Anti-inflammatory supplements	70.1	78.9	55.8
Sedatives	8.3	8.6	8.0
Erythropoietin	1.0	0.4	1.8
Anabolic agents	0.7	0.4	1.2

consume the proper amount of calories and nutrients. However, they should not be considered as replacement for a good diet.

Today, the supplement industry is an international market worth billions of dollars. According to the estimates of a *Nutrition Business Journal* report, the global supplement market stood at USD 104 billion in 2013 [5]. Strongly outpacing other major consumer health categories, sport supplements broke the USD 10 billion retail value sales mark in 2014 [6]. North America holds the largest market share for sport supplements, followed by Europe and Asia Pacific [6].

Most data reported in the literature show that nearly half of all athletes use supplements, with wide variation between different sports and between athletes of differing performance levels, ages, and cultural backgrounds. For example, a high percentage of Canadian Olympic athletes were found to consume dietary supplements at the Atlanta (69%) and Sydney (74%) Olympic Games [7]. In some sports, such as strength and power sports, supplement intake is so common it is perceived as the norm.

Also, individuals engaged in recreational sports or other fitness pursuits are much interested in the advantages of taking supplements.

In 2012, an Italian survey from UISP (Unione Italiana Sport per Tutti) with a grant from the Istituto Superiore di Sanità (ISS) investigated the consumption of ergogenic substances and food supplements in a group of adolescents and adults attending gyms and fitness centers (n = 451) [8]. Results (table 1) pointed out that vitamins were the most used supplements in both males and females (53.4% of individuals declared to have consumed them in the last year). Proteins and amino acid derivatives (mainly creatine) have been used by 12.4% of the individuals, with men consuming more than double the amount of women, probably due to the fact that males are more interested in enlarging muscle mass [8].

Interestingly, 77% of individuals interviewed met the costs for substances listed in table 1. The percentage of minors who paid for these products was higher than thought and comparable to the other age classes. The difference among age classes consisted in the volume of expenditure per year, which increased with age (EUR 46.7 for young

Table 2. The function of supplements according to athletes (adapted from Maughan et al. [10])

Objectives	Substances
Muscle growth and repair	Protein powder and hydrolysate, amino acids, essential amino acids, HMB
Fat reduction	Pyruvate, caffeine, carnitine
Exercise metabolism	Carbohydrate, caffeine, bicarbonate, creatine
Promoting recovery	Whole-protein powders, protein isolates, hydrosylates, protein carbohydrate bars and drinks, ginseng
General health	Vitamins, minerals, evening primrose oil
Immune function	Echinacea, antioxidants, zinc, lycopene
CNS stimulation	Taurine, caffeine, guarana
Meal replacement	Liquid meals, sports bars, carbohydrate gels
Fluid and electrolyte solution	Sports drinks, electrolyte supplements

people aged 14–18 years and EUR 174 for those aged ≥26 years). About 10% of the sample declared to spend more than EUR 250 per year [8].

The regulation of supplements and sport foods is a contentious area. There is no universal system of regulation, and countries differ in their approach and practice. According to the European Commission (EC), a food supplement is a concentrated source of nutrients or other substances with a nutritional or physiological effect whose purpose is to supplement the normal diet [9]. They are marketed in dose form; i.e. as pills, tablets, capsules, powders, and liquids in measured small units. The regulation clearly states that supplements may be used to correct nutritional deficiencies or maintain an adequate intake of certain nutrients. However, in many cases, their sale and use are not completely in line with the spirit of the regulation.

Athletes should always consider the issue of efficacy, safety, and legality associated with supplements before using them. However, the number of products is enormous while the correct information is limited. In many cases, 'evidence' is related to insufficient data or low-quality studies. Furthermore, studies are often not relevant to real-life sport events; for example, laboratory studies of cycle ergometer performance, treadmill running, and isometric strength may have little relevance to competitive athletes. Similarly, results could not apply to all different subpopulation groups. As a consequence, the decision to use a supplement is frequently extrapolated from inappropriate data rather than clear-cut evidence. Maughan et al. [10] categorized some supplements according to athletes' belief of target function (table 2).

Sport Supplement Efficacy

Sport nutrition professionals need to know how to evaluate the scientific value of articles and advertisements on nutritional practices and supplements in order to distinguish scientific evidence from the marketing hype.

Table 3. Factors to consider when assessing a research paper on sport supplements (adapted from Braun et al. [11])

Factors	Considerations
Participants	Are they similar to the athletes/sport practitioners the supplement is suggested to? Are they comparable for age, gender, and training status?
Type of performance test	Is the test valid and reliable?
Control of the study	Is the study well controlled? Does it account for diet, training, and sleep?
Study design	Is the study placebo controlled and double blind? Was the statistical power correctly calculated? Is the study acute or chronic? Which is the supplement ingestion mode/vehicle?
Supplement	Have the active components been analyzed and quantified? Has the supplement been tested for contaminants, particularly banned substances?
Funding source	Has funding source been correctly declared?

When assessing the ergogenic value of a dietary supplement the theoretical rationale behind the supplement and the scientific evidence supporting its ergogenic value must be carefully examined.

According to the International Society of Sports Nutrition (ISSN) [1], there are three main questions to ask when evaluating the potential ergogenic value of a supplement:

(1) Does the theory make sense?

(2) Is there any scientific evidence supporting the ergogenic value?

(3) Is the supplement safe and legal?

As regards the second question, some important factors have to be considered when assessing research papers on sport supplements (summarized in table 3). Among the most critical aspects, the measurement of the performance-enhancing effect is still open to debate, as many variables concur and thus make it difficult to find the measurable outcome strictly correlating to the performance outcome. This aspect is even more complicated for sports where performance is not necessarily determined by physiological outcomes (e.g. basketball and tennis).

Four categories of supplements can be identified based on the actual level of scientific evidence [1]:

(1) Apparently effective (most research finds them to be effective and safe);

(2) Possibly effective (supplements of which initial research has supported the theoretical rationale in consumption, yet further studies are required);

(3) Too early to tell (supplements with insufficient scientific evidence to support their efficacy);

Table 4. Categorization of some sport supplements based on the available literature (adapted from Kreider et al. [1])

	Sport foods	Performance-enhancing supplements	Muscle building and repair supplements
Apparently effective	Carbohydrate- or protein-based drinks, powders, bars Carbohydrate-electrolyte-based drinks, powders, bars	Caffeine Creatine Sodium bicarbonate Sodium citrate	
Possibly effective		Amino acids Essential amino acids Branched-chain amino acids HMB	Branched-chain amino acids Essential amino acids HMB Leucine
Too early to tell		Medium-chain triglycerides	α-Ketoglutarate
Apparently ineffective		Glutamine Ribose Inosine Chromium L-Carnitine	Glutamine Boron Chromium Conjugated linoleic acids Isoflavones

(4) Apparently ineffective (supplements for which the rationale behind their consumption is low and research identifies them as ineffective).

Similarly, the *APRID* framework [11], devised by Braun, Currell, and Stear, divided supplements into five categories based on a risk-benefit analysis from scientific research and clinical dietetic practice:

A: Acceptable (scientific research has shown a clear performance or health benefit);

P: Physiological (there is a physiological rationale but the performance or health outcome is unclear);

R: Research (there is practitioner-based evidence);

I: Ineffective (there is no clear performance or health benefit);

D: Disallowed (products banned or at high risk).

On the basis of these proposals, a categorization of common supplements used for sports and physical activity is reported in table 4.

It is also important to consider that, generally speaking, supporting evidence-based claims have become more challenging as regulators seek science behind claim specifications. The review of dossiers promoting health claims carried out by the European Food Safety Authority (EFSA) has reduced the marketing of health claim benefits of dietary supplements in Europe. The intention was not to obstruct the supplement market but rather to enforce scientific substantiation and regulatory standards. EFSA's Scientific Opinion on some approved claims for sport supplements are summarized in table 5. It is essential to highlight that the positive opinions were substantiated by taking the totality of the available pertinent scientific data into account and evaluating the evidence. In particular, the evidence should demonstrate the extent to which:

(1) The effect is relevant for human health;

(2) A cause-effect relationship is established between the consumption of the nutrient/substance/food or food category and the claimed effect in humans (such as the strength, consistency, specificity, dose-response, and biological plausibility of the relationship);

(3) The effect is shown on a study group representative of the target population;

(4) The quantity of the food and the pattern of consumption required to obtain the claimed effect could reasonably be achieved as part of a balanced diet.

Sport Supplement Specificity

As already mentioned, specificity of action is an important factor to consider when deciding to take a supplement. First of all, the use of a supplement should be planned on the basis of the kind of sport and the performance level of the athletes. For example, although sodium bicarbonate may improve performance in middle-distance running (400–5,000 m) [17], there is no reason to think that there will be any benefit to jumpers or throwers. Furthermore, data from well-trained athletes cannot be applied to sport practitioners without knowing their physical conditions and food habits before and during competitions.

For some supplements, the nutritional status can affect the individual response. In fact, it is increasingly recognized that individual athletes will respond differently to vitamin or mineral supplements: the athlete who suffers from a deficiency is likely to show a benefit in response to a period of supplementation, but the well-nourished athlete is unlikely to see an improvement in health or performance when taking the same supplement [10].

Differences could be present also according to age, gender as well as structural, hormonal, and metabolic characteristics. Regarding age, many young boys and girls eager to improve their performance are attracted by supplements. The results of the National Health Interview Survey [18], which was published in 2012, revealed that more than 1.2 million American adolescents (1.6% of adolescents with an average age of 10.8 years) were taking supplements for sport performance. A longitudinal Australian study, including more than 900 young (12- to 17-year-old) athletes competing at elite junior level, showed that about 4% of them took performance-enhancing drugs and supplements [19]. Supplement use tends to differ across genders for prevalence, types of supplements, as well as reasons for use. In this regard, males tend to put more emphasis on the athletic performance-enhancing effects whereas females tend to be more concerned with the health benefits. In a study by Ziegler et

Table 5. EFSA Panel Scientific Opinion on the substantiation of health claims related to some supplements of nutrients/substances (in italics) and physical performance

Claim	Condition of use of the claim	Health relationship
Carbohydrate-electrolyte solutions [12]		
Carbohydrate-electrolyte solutions contribute to the maintenance of endurance performance during prolonged endurance exercise	In order to bear the claim, carbohydrate-electrolyte solutions should contain 80–350 kcal/l from carbohydrates, and at least 75% of the energy should be derived from carbohydrates which induce a high glycemic response, such as glucose, glucose polymers and sucrose; in addition, these beverages should contain between 20 mM (460 mg/l) and 50 mM (1,150 mg/l) of sodium, and have an osmolality of 200–330 mOsm/kg water	Maintenance of endurance performance
Carbohydrate-electrolyte solutions enhance the absorption of water during physical exercise		Enhancement of water absorption during exercise
Carbohydrates [13]		
Carbohydrates contribute to the recovery of normal muscle function (contraction) after highly intensive and/or long-lasting physical exercise leading to muscle fatigue and the depletion of glycogen stores in skeletal muscles	The claim may be used only for food which provides carbohydrates which are metabolized by humans (excluding polyols); the effect is obtained with the consumption of carbohydrates, from all sources, at a total intake of 4 g/kg body weight, at doses, within the first 4 h and not later than 6 h following highly intensive and/or long-lasting physical exercise leading to muscle fatigue and the depletion of glycogen stores in skeletal muscle; the claim may be used only for foods intended for adults who have performed highly intensive and/or long-lasting physical exercise leading to muscle fatigue and the depletion of glycogen stores in skeletal muscle	
Creatine [14]		
Creatine increases physical performance in successive bursts of short-term, high-intensity exercise	The claim may be used only for food which provides a daily intake of 3 g of creatine; in order to bear the claim, information shall be given to the consumer that the beneficial effect is obtained with a daily intake of 3 g of creatine; the claim may be used only for foods targeting adults performing high-intensity exercise	Increase in physical performance during short-term, high-intensity, repeated exercise bouts
Vitamin C [15]		
Vitamin C helps to maintain the normal function of the immune system during and after intense physical exercise	The claim may be used only for food which provides a daily intake of 200 mg of vitamin C; in order to bear the claim, information shall be given to the consumer that the beneficial effect is obtained with a daily intake of 200 mg in addition to the recommended daily intake of vitamin C	Function of the immune system during and after extreme physical exercise

Table 5. Continued

Claim	Condition of use of the claim	Health relationship
Caffeine [16]		
Caffeine contributes to an increase in endurance performance	In order to obtain the claimed effect, caffeine should be consumed at doses of 3 mg/kg body weight 1 h prior to exercise; the target population is adults performing endurance exercise	Increase in physical performance during short-term endurance activities
Caffeine contributes to an increase in endurance capacity		Supports exercise performance (reduction in perceived exertion, improve time to exhaustion and exercise capacity)
Caffeine contributes to a reduction in the rated perceived exertion/effort during exercise	In order to obtain the claimed effect, caffeine should be consumed at doses of 4 mg/kg body weight 1 h prior to exercise; the target population is adults performing endurance exercise	Supports exercise performance (reduction in perceived exertion, improve time to exhaustion and exercise capacity) and reduces perception of effort

al. [20] on young elite figure skaters emerged that females consumed multivitamin/mineral supplements most frequently (83%), followed by herbal supplements (48%), and multivitamin-only supplements (42%). These products could be categorized as health-related supplements, where males also used multivitamin/mineral (61%) and herbal supplements (44%), but consumed protein bars (38%), protein powders (15%), amino acid powders (8%), and creatine (3%) more frequently than their female counterparts, confirming that males tend to use supplements claiming a more ergogenic effect. The only exception to this is that females (35%) consumed energy drinks and bars slightly more frequently than males (33%) [20].

Finally, athletes should also avoid to use supplements in an inappropriate way, taking them at the wrong time or at too high or too low doses.

Ergogenic Aids: The Proof of Concept

In the present section, the efficacy of some of the most popular supplements used to enhance physical performance will be discussed. Particular attention will be focused on: amino acids and their derivatives [e.g. creatine and β-hydroxy-β-methylbutyrate (HMB)], caffeine, caffeinated energy drinks, and antioxidants (e.g. vitamins and glutathione).

Effect of Creatine on Sport Performance

Creatine is one of the most popular natural supplements formed by arginine and glycine. Creatine is produced endogenously in the liver, kidneys, and pancreas (up to 1 g/day), or obtained through the diet (at about 1 g/day) [21]. In humans, the majority of creatine is in two forms: phosphorylated (up to 60% of the stores) or free (up to 40% of the stores). A total of 95% of creatine is stored in skeletal muscles, in particular in fast-twitch type II fibers [21]. Cells use phosphocreatine as donor of phosphate to produce adenosine triphosphate, which is useful as energy substrate for the contraction of skeletal muscles [21]. A 2013 National Collegiate Athletic Association (NCAA) survey study reported that 14% of student athletes, especially wrestlers, use creatine [22]. A 2003 meta-analysis of 22 studies showed that although creatine supplementation was more effective on predominantly anaerobic intermittent exercise, there was some evidence of its positive effects also on endurance activities [23]. However, the ergogenic potential on aerobic endurance exercise diminished as the duration of the activity increased over 150 s, possibly due to a change in substrate utilization. A more recent meta-analysis of 60 randomized controlled trials on the effects of creatine on lower-limb strength performance showed that supplementation is effective in lower-limb strength performance for exercises lasting less than 3 min, independent of population characteristics, training protocols, and supplementary doses and duration [24]. Creatine ingestion increases the total creatine content in human muscles by approximately 15–20% following ingestion of 20 g per day for 4–5 days, but also by ingestion of 3 g per day over a period of 1 month [14]. Long-term creatine supplementation (e.g. 4–12 weeks) in combination with training appears to increase muscle mass and strength as a result of an improved ability to perform high-intensity exercise via increased creatine phosphate availability [14, 25]. Collectively, in spite of a few controversial results [26–28], creatine supplementation combined with resistance training seems to be able to amplify performance enhancement to the maximum and endurance strength as well muscle hypertrophy. Based on these data, in a 2007 position statement, the ISSN declared that the use of creatine as a nutritional supplement within established guidelines is safe, and effectively improves anaerobic capacity, strength, and lean body mass in conjunction with training [25].

Similarly, in weighing the evidence from short- and long-term creatine supplementation studies, EFSA adopted a favorable opinion about the role of creatine in increasing physical performance during short-term, high-intensity, repeated exercise bouts. In order to obtain the claimed effect, 3 g of creatine should be consumed daily by adults performing high-intensity exercise. On the contrary, EFSA rejected the claims about the endurance capacity and endurance performance since a cause-effect relationship has not been established yet [14].

Creatine supplementation has also been shown to improve recovery from injury, muscle damage, and oxidative stress induced by exercise. Bassit et al. [29] observed a decrease in several markers of muscle damage in a pilot study performed in a group of 4 athletes supplemented with 20 g/day plus 50 g maltodextrin during a 5-day period prior to an iron man competition. Cooke et al. [30] observed a positive effect of a prior (0.3 g/day/kg body weight) loading and a postmaintenance protocol (0.1 g/day/kg body weight) to attenuate the loss of strength and muscle damage after an acute supramaximal eccentric resistance training session in young males. Rahimi [31] documented a significant increase in athletic performance, and a significant reduction in oxidative stress, induced by a single bout of resistance exercise following 7-day supplementation of creatine monohydrate (20 g/day) in a group of male athletes. The above investigations indicate that creatine supplementation can attenuate muscle damage induced by a prolonged endurance training session and act as an antioxidant agent. However, further studies should be performed in order to come to any conclusions.

Role of Caffeine and Caffeinated Energy Drinks on Physical Performance
Caffeine is a fat-soluble molecule naturally present in many foods and drinks (i.e. coffee, tea, and chocolate) and added to many energy drinks and sport food. The content varies widely in relation to the quality and variety of foods (from 5–10 mg for 60 g of chocolate up to 200 mg for a cup of espresso) [32]. Typically, caffeine-containing energy drinks contain from 25 to 250 mg of caffeine in various forms, from alkaloid caffeine to caffeine-containing plant extracts [32]. Caffeine is the most used psychoactive substance in the world; it is estimated that the daily intake is around 200 mg. Caffeine intake from foods such as soft drinks, chocolate, gum, and candy in children and adolescents may reach up to 16 mg/day for children aged 7–8 years, 24 mg/day for those aged 9–10 years, and up to 37.4 mg/day for adolescents/young adults (18 years old) [33]. Most caffeine intake among the young comes from soda. Once absorbed, caffeine is metabolized in the liver to paraxanthine (84%), theobromine (12%), and theophylline (4%); these substances maintain in part the biological activities of caffeine [32]. Recognized as a stimulant, caffeine is used mainly to improve cognitive function and physical performance. For this reason, it has long been considered a doping substance and banned from sports competition until 2004 [32]. Actually, caffeine is commonly used by athletes because of its reported ergogenic effects. Three mechanisms have been suggested by which caffeine may improve physical performance: (1) by increasing the mobilization of intracellular calcium; (2) by increasing free fatty acid oxidation, and (3) by serving as an adenosine receptor antagonist in the central nervous system. The last seems to be the mechanism most likely involved in the ergogenic effect, as recently documented [34, 35]. The link of caffeine to the A1 receptor generates an increase in intracellular cyclic AMP levels, followed by increases in the concentration of cytoplasmic calcium and the activation of the Na^+/K^+ pump. Through this mechanism, caffeine may modulate central fatigue and influence ratings of perceived exertion, perceived pain, and levels of vigor, all of which may lead to performance improvements [32, 34, 35]. Most of the ergogenic effects have been observed following the administration of low caffeine doses (3 mg/kg body weight, about 200 mg for a 70-kg individual). Acute doses higher than 9 mg/kg did not show any

performance gain, and, in many cases, the administration of high doses induced several adverse effects such as palpitations, headache, weakness, shivering, and anxiety [32, 36].

In a recent review, the analysis of 24 studies showed that the administration of 2–5 mg/kg caffeine prior to performance-based exercise enhanced sport performances by increasing exercise duration and by improving completion time at about 3.6% [37]. The results are in accordance with the findings reviewed by Ganio et al. [35] that documented an improvement (about 3.2%) of athletic performance following the administration of similar doses of caffeine. Conversely, in a sedentary state, caffeine has shown to impair insulin action and, thus, glycemic regulation. A position stand from the ISSN summarized the effects of caffeine on exercise performance [36]. Briefly, caffeine is effective for enhancing sport performance in trained athletes when consumed in low/moderate dosages (about 3–6 mg/kg body weight), while no effect has been observed for high dosages (≥9 mg/kg body weight). Caffeine is ergogenic for sustained maximal endurance exercise, especially for time trial performance and for enhancing vigilance during bouts of extended exhaustive exercise. Moreover, a supplementation with caffeine is beneficial for high-intensity exercise, especially for those that are categorized by intermittent activity within a period of prolonged duration, but the effects of caffeine on diuresis during exercise and on strength-power performance remain unclear [36].

Most frequently, athletes consume caffeine in energy drinks. It is important to consider that these products are extremely popular not only in adults but also in adolescents. Analysis of the recent literature reveals that frequent or excessive intake of caloric sport drinks and caffeinated energy drinks can induce tachycardia, cardiac dysrhythmias, hypertension, and heart failure, and substantially increase the risk of overweight or obesity in children and adolescents [38]. Regarding the potential ergogenic effects of caffeine-containing energy drinks, an analysis of the 7 studies reported in literature reviewed by Ganio et al. [35] confirmed enhanced performance. However, the results were highly variable depending on the beverages consumed, the range of caffeine doses administered, the timing of ingestion, as well as the type, intensity, and duration of physical activity performed. It is documented that the intake of a sugar-free caffeine-containing energy drink (3 mg/kg) is able to enhance sport performances in soccer, rugby, basketball, and badminton players. The improvements were related to jump height, power output, distance covered, running speed, and the number of sprints performed within a game [39–44]. In a recent position statement, the ISSN concluded that the consumption of energy drinks (containing approximately 2 mg/kg body weight of caffeine) 45–60 min prior to anaerobic/resistance exercise may improve upper- and lower-body total lifting volume. However, no effect on repeated high-intensity sprint exercise or on agility performance was observed [45]. On the contrary, the same energy drinks consumed 10–40 min prior to aerobic exercise improved cycling and running performance in both trained cyclists and recreationally active participants [45].

Similarly, evaluating the evidence from short- and long-term caffeine supplementation, EFSA adopted a favorable opinion about the role of caffeine to increase endurance performance and endurance capacity. The Panel considers that in order to obtain the claimed effect in adults performing endurance exercise, caffeine should be consumed at doses of 3 mg/kg body weight 1 h prior to exercise. Moreover, the Panel concluded that a cause-effect relationship has also been established between the consumption of caffeine and a reduction in the rated perceived exertion/effort during exercise. In order to obtain this effect, caffeine should be consumed at doses of 4 mg/kg body weight 1 h prior to exercise [16]. On the contrary, EFSA rejected the claim related to an increase in physical performance during short-term high-intensity exercise since a cause-effect relationship has not been established yet [16].

It is important to highlight that the potential ergogenic effects of caffeine and other stimulant substances contained in energy drinks on children and adolescents have not been investigated in more detail. Few recent studies reported an improvement in physical performance in junior tennis players [46] and adolescent basketball players [41]. Although the US Food and Drug Administration limits caffeine content in soft drinks, which are categorized as food, there is no such regulation for energy drinks, which are classified as dietary supplements. For most children, adolescents, and young adults, safe levels of caffeine consumption have not been established.

Role of β-Hydroxy-β-Methylbutyrate on Sport Performance

HMB is a metabolite of the branched-chain amino acid leucine and its keto acid α-ketoisocaproate. A 2013 NCAA survey study reported a 0.2% rate of use among student athletes [22]. HMB is believed to attenuate protein breakdown after workouts and it is extensively used by athletes and bodybuilders in order to increase strength, muscle mass, and exercise performance. Three of the possible advocated mechanisms involved in the improvement in sport performance are: (1) enhancement of sarcolemmal integrity via cytosolic cholesterol, (2) inhibition of protein degradation via proteasomes, and (3) increase of protein synthesis via the mTOR (mammalian target of rapamycin) pathway [47]. Recent studies suggested additional possible mechanisms for its physiological effects. These include decreased cell apoptosis and enhanced cell survival, increased proliferation, differentiation, and fusion via the mitogen-activated protein kinase/extracellular signal-regulated kinase and phosphatidylinositol 3-kinase/Akt pathways, and enhanced insulin-like growth factor-1 transcription [48].

The effect of HMB supplementation on sport performance has been studied in a variety of anaerobic and aerobic training conditions [49]. However, it is difficult to compare results due to differences in the dosing schedules and amounts of HMB, training levels of participants, and performance outcomes. Several studies supported the efficacy of HMB supplementation to improve sport performance by enhancing recovery [50, 51], lean body mass [50, 52], strength [53], power [54], and aerobic performance [55] in athletes. However, other studies documented a more evident improvement in untrained subjects with respect to athletes [56–59]. For example, Palisin and Stacy [59] reported that HMB supplementation determined gains in strength and lean body mass in patients with wasting syndromes. Rowlands and Thomson [58] analyzed the effectiveness of HMB supplementation (range 1.5–6.0 g/day) on strength, body composition, and muscle damage in trained and untrained young men. The results documented a trivial effect of HMB supplementation on all muscle strength outcomes in trained men and benefits on lower-body and average leg strength in untrained men [58]. In a recent systematic review, Molfino et al. [56] concluded that the usual dose of 3 g/day of HBM may be routinely recommended to maintain or improve muscle mass and function in young and elderly untrained subjects and in those affected by chronic diseases.

It is against this background, therefore, that official statements and positions from scientific organizations and institutions are still controversial. A position stand from the ISSN provided recommendations on the optimization of the effects of HBM on body composition, strength, power, and aerobic performance across varying levels of age, sex, and training status [47]. Briefly, the ISSN stated that HMB can be used to enhance recovery by attenuating exercise-induced skeletal muscle damage in trained and untrained populations, and that a supplementation appears to be most effective when performed for 2 weeks prior to an exercise bout. Moreover, a daily supplementation (38 mg/kg of body mass) should enhance skeletal muscle hypertrophy, strength, and power in both untrained and trained subjects when the appropriate exercise prescription is utilized. Lastly, HMB has been demonstrated to increase lean body mass and functionality in elderly, sedentary populations, and, in conjunction with a structured exercise program, may result in greater declines in fat mass [47].

On the other hand, EFSA ruled negatively about the capacity of HMB, alone or in combination with α-ketoisocaproate, to reduce muscle tissue damage during exercise, to increase lean body mass, muscle strength, endurance performance, and skeletal muscle tissue repair, and for faster recovery from muscle fatigue after exercise, since a cause-effect relationship has not been established [60]. In fact, data provided are still limited and inconsistent, and no evidence for a mechanism by which HMB could exert the claimed effect was provided.

For all these reasons, HMB is included in the list of 'apparently effective' substances reported in table 4.

Role of Dietary Antioxidants on Sport Performance

During physical activity, metabolism, muscle activity, and oxygen utilization tend to increase resulting in the generation of reactive oxygen species (ROS) and nitrogen species that can alter cell structure and function, and contribute to muscle damage, immune dysfunction, tiredness, and fatigue. Antioxidant supplements may have direct or indirect effects on exercise performance [61]. Direct effects could involve the reduction in muscle fatigue at the level of contractile function, while indirect effects could include enhancement of training, reduction in physiological stressors, or improvement in the ability to recover from training. However, there are many doubts regarding the advantages and disadvantages of using antioxidants to improve physical performance. The effects of a wide range of dietary antioxidants on sport performance will be summarized.

Vitamin C

Vitamin C is a water-soluble vitamin that plays an important role in collagen and cortisol syntheses and as a scavenger of free radicals. Therefore, supplementation with vitamin C could enhance athletic performance counteracting ROS production, reducing muscle damage, and delaying onset of muscle soreness. The role of a vitamin C supplementation on sport performance has been investigated in many trials [62–64]. The majority of studies have attempted to examine the longer-term effects of vitamin C supplementation instead of an acute effect. While the earliest studies appeared promising, recent and more rigorous trials do not seem to support the ergogenic role of vitamin C [65–67]. A recent review by Braakhuis [63] showed that high doses of vitamin C (>1 g/day) seem to impair sport performance by reducing training-induced adaptations in athletes, while physiological doses (at about 200 mg/day) have shown to be sufficient to induce a reduction in oxidative stress and provide beneficial effects on athletes without impairing training adaptations. The most important beneficial effects observed in exercise training are the attenuation of exercise-induced bronchoconstriction and asthma, the decrease in muscle damage as well as the maintenance of normal functions of the immune system during and after extreme physical exercise. This latter function was also recognized by EFSA that authorized the claim 'Contributes to maintain the normal function of the immune system during and after intense physical exercise' for concentrations of vitamin C of 200 mg/day in addition to the usual diet [15].

In conclusion, considering current data, administration of nonphysiological doses of vitamin C in healthy athletes seems not to be suggested because of the possibility to impair adaptation to regular exercise.

Vitamin E

Vitamin E is a well-recognized, fat-soluble vitamin with antioxidant activity able to protect cells from oxidative damage, and, thus, it should be able to counteract an oxidative stress condition by improving physical performance. However, data from human intervention studies are quite controversial. A recent review summarized the main results deriving from acute and chronic vitamin E supplementation in different sport performances [68]. Only 1 of 12 studies was an acute study [69]. The intake of a single dose of carbohydrate-protein beverage fortified with vitamin E (20 mg during exercise and 133 mg after exercise) seemed to confer performance benefits and attenuate muscle damage in athletes after exercise [69]. On the contrary, studies on chronic intake of vitamin E (100–300 mg/day for 1–6 months) showed impairment in physical performance rather than an ergogenic effect [68]. No effect was observed on performance during standard exercise tests and cardiorespiratory fitness tests, while a feeble effect in the modulation of muscle contraction and attenuation of muscle damage was documented. Altitude was found to increase oxidative stress and reduce red blood cell deformability in climbers [70, 71]. A supplementation with 300 mg vitamin E per day for 4 weeks at an altitude of 5,000 m showed to offset the impairment by maintaining red blood cells deformability in climbers [70, 71]. However, this evidence was only observed in two old studies performed in subjects exposed to extreme conditions and merits further investigations.

In conclusion, the evidence available suggests that the daily intake of doses of vitamin E higher than recommended daily allowances (15 mg/day) should be avoided by athletes. More studies in humans are needed to clarify the effects of vitamin E supplementation on sport performance in athletes.

Glutathione and N-Acetyl Cysteine

Glutathione (GSH) is a tripeptide synthesized from cysteine, glycine, and glutamate. It is an endogenous antioxidant that acts as scavenger against ROS and as cofactor of phase II antioxidant enzymes, such as glutathione peroxidase and glutathione S-transferase. Moreover, GSH plays a crucial role in recycling several antioxidants, including vitamin C and E radicals [61, 68]. The biosynthesis of GSH, by way of the γ-glutamyl cycle, is important for maintaining its homeostasis and normal redox status. N-acetylcysteine (NAC), a water-soluble precursor of GSH, is one of the antioxidant supplements commonly used in exercise training by several athletes. The effects of NAC supplementation against oxidative stress in athletes and its capability to improve sport performance has been investigated in some small acute and chronic studies [68].

In an acute study, intravenous infusion of NAC (125 mg/kg/h for 15 min and then 25 mg/kg/h for 20 min before and throughout exercise) was performed to evaluate the effect on fatigue during prolonged, submaximal exercise in endurance athletes. The results showed that NAC administration improved performance in well-trained individuals, with enhanced muscle cysteine and GSH availability a likely mechanism [72]. In another acute study on 8 well-trained subjects, the authors showed, using the same experimental conditions (intravenous NAC infusion of 125 mg/kg/h for 15 min and then 25 mg/kg/h for 20 min before and throughout exercise), an attenuation in muscle fatigue and reduction in oxidative stress [73]. A significant reduction in respiratory muscle fatigue was also observed following an acute oral dose of NAC (1,800 mg, 45 min prior to a 30-min discontinuous exercise) in a group of 8 subjects during heavy exercise [73].

Regarding the impact of chronic NAC supplementation, the results are controversial. Seven-day administration of 2,400 mg of NAC decreased muscle fatigue in a group of 9 untrained healthy men following maximal exercise [74]. In a more recent study, a 9-day oral NAC supplementation (1,200 mg/day) improved cycling performance via an improved redox balance and promoted adaptive processes in a group of 10 well-trained athletes undergoing strenuous physical training [75]. On the contrary, a 7-day oral NAC supplementation (100 mg/kg body weight) in 9 well-trained male cyclists altered substrate metabolism and muscle fiber type recruitment during high-intensity interval exercise with detrimental effects on time trial performance [76].

In conclusion, the ergogenic role of NAC is inconsistent and quite controversial. Most of the positive observations were detected in very small groups of subjects (max. 10 athletes) and should be corroborated in larger cohorts. Moreover, recent findings on cellular pathways report that NAC supplementation may impair intrinsic responses and recovery of muscles [61, 77]. Thus, further researches are necessary.

Ubiquinones

Ubiquinones are lipid-soluble antioxidants able to prevent lipid peroxidation and play an important role in vitamin E recycling [61]. Coenzyme Q_{10} (CoQ_{10}) represents the most predominant form of ubiquinones in humans. Some studies documented a positive relationship between exercise capacity and CoQ_{10} plasma concentrations in physically active males. Díaz-Castro et al. [78] reported that a 3-day CoQ_{10} supplementation (5 capsules of 30 mg of CoQ_{10}) decreased oxidative stress and muscle damage in a group of runners before a constant run (50 km) that combined several degrees of high effort (mountain run and ultra-endurance) in permanent climbing. In another study, a 12-day CoQ_{10} supplementation (300 mg/day CoQ_{10}) reduced oxidative stress markers and improved physical performance of young swimmers by increasing maximal treadmill time [79]. Two older intervention studies reported that 30-day supplementation with 100 mg of CoQ_{10} per day was able to increase endurance capacity and/or endurance performance in sedentary people and athletes [80, 81]. In contrast, some studies failed to demonstrate an ergogenic property for CoQ_{10}, while another study found impaired performance in high-intensity endurance tests after supplementation with CoQ_{10} [82].

In conclusion, current data regarding CoQ_{10} supplementation during exercise training are inconsistent. EFSA rejected the claims about the role of CoQ_{10} in the improvement in physical endurance and performance since a cause-effect relationship has not been established [83].

Lipoic Acids

α-Lipoic acid is an endogenous thiol and cofactor of α-dehydrogenase complexes. In cells, lipoic acid is reduced to dihydrolipoic acid, an important agent in vitamin C recycling during oxidative stress [84]. Supplementation with α-lipoic acid enhances muscle phosphocreatine levels and muscle total creatine concentrations, and consequently has a potentially enhancing effect on short-term exercise [82]. However, its effects on exercise performance are unknown. A recent study performed on a group of 16 healthy young males reported that the intake of α-lipoic acid (1,200 mg daily for 10 days prior to exercise) was able to reduce oxidative stress, enhance erythropoietin release, and reduce muscle damage after running eccentric exercise [85]. Zembron-Lacny et al. [86] documented that α-lipoic acid supplementation (600 mg/day, for

8 days) was able to modulate a proantioxidant response to the muscle-damaging exercise in trained men.

In conclusion, there are insufficient data to document a role of α-lipoic acid supplementation in physical performance.

Polyphenols and Polyphenol-Rich Foods

Polyphenols are a big family of bioactive compounds widely distributed in whole plant foods. Despite their rapid and low absorption in the human body, these compounds have potent antioxidant properties and are involved in the modulation of several important cell signaling pathways. Numerous in vitro and in vivo studies documented the capacity of polyphenols, in a variety of forms and doses, to positively affect markers of oxidative stress [87]. In this regard, recent studies performed in our laboratories showed that the consumption of polyphenol-rich foods, such as blueberries, counteracted endothelial dysfunction and reduced oxidative DNA damage in healthy subjects and in those with cardiovascular risk factors [88–90]. However, the role of polyphenols and polyphenol-rich foods on physical performance has not been investigated in more detail. Chang et al. [91] reported that consuming a high-polyphenol diet (200 g of purple sweet potato leaves per day) for 7 days can modulate antioxidant status and decrease exercise-induced oxidative damage and proinflammatory cytokine secretion in healthy untrained young men after a running exercise. McAnulty et al. [92] showed that the administration of 150 g of blueberries per day for 6 weeks and a portion of 375 g of blueberries 1 h prior to 2.5 h of running at about 72% maximal oxygen consumption significantly decreased serum levels of free radicals in athletes in a hot environment. Lafay et al. [93] documented that a 30-day supplementation with 400 mg of grape extract, containing oligomeric proanthocyanidins, per day enhanced physical performance in elite male athletes during physical exercise. A recent meta-analysis of 11 different studies on the role of quercetin supplementation on endurance performance showed that, although an improvement in endurance exercise performance and endurance exercise capacity was observed following supplementation (median dose 1,000 mg/day), the changes were not significantly different from placebo [94]. Recently, Yarahmadi et al. [95] reported that 6-week supplementation with anthocyanin pills (100 mg/day) was able to improve some indices of exercise performance in a group of athletes.

Concerning the use of polyphenol-rich juice (including pomegranate, chokeberry, and cherry juice) as supplements in exercise studies, the evidence cannot support the role of these products in the improvement in endurance performance [68].

An increasing interest has been noted towards the effects of polyphenols and polyphenol-rich foods in the context of muscle damage and performance recovery after muscle microdamage. In comparison to endurance performance studies, trials on this topic seem more promising. For example, Pilaczynska-Szczesniak et al. [96] reported that the consumption of 150 ml of chokeberry juice per day (providing 34 mg of anthocyanins) for 30 days was able to limit the exercise-induced oxidative damage by enhancing the endogenous antioxidant defense system. Bowtell et al. [97] showed that the consumption of a cherry juice (60 ml/day containing 300 mg of anthocyanins) for 7 days before and 48 h after intensive exercise improved the recovery of isometric muscle strength and attenuated oxidative damage, induced by the damaging exercise, in a group of 10 well-trained male overnight-fasted athletes. Trombold et al. [98] documented that a 7-day supplementation with pomegranate juice (providing approximatively 200 mg of anthocyanins and 60 mg of ellagic acid) attenuated weakness and reduced soreness of the elbow flexor but not of knee extensor muscles in a group of resistance-trained men after eccentric exercise.

In conclusion, polyphenols can have beneficial effects on sport performance by decreasing oxidative stress; these effects can be obtained by introducing an amount of polyphenols easily reached through the diet (e.g. consumption of 5 or more servings of fruit and vegetables) without the need of specific ergogenic products. However, their role in the modulation of endurance performance is not clearly understood and should be further investigated. Preliminary evidence suggests to address the research on recovery from muscle microdamage in order to gain better insight.

Other Substances

In addition to the supplements previously described that showed some positive ergogenic effect, there are several substances that lack scientific rationale, or have been clearly demonstrated to be ineffective in promoting an ergogenic effect. This is, for example, the case of glutamine and isoflavones.

Glutamine

L-Glutamine, the most abundant non-essential amino acid in the body, has shown to increase cell volume, and stimulate protein and glycogen synthesis [99, 100]. Theoretically, glutamine supplementation should increase muscle mass and enhance gains in strength during training. However, there is no compelling evidence to support L-glutamine supplementation as a potential ergogenic product in terms of increasing lean body mass or muscular performance, or repair skeletal muscle tissue in adults performing strenuous exercise [101].

Isoflavones

Isoflavones are nonsteroidal phytoestrogens that showed promising results in preventing declines in bone mass in postmenopausal women [102]. Recently, it has been theorized that two isoflavone extracts (ipriflavone and methoxyisoflavone) can increase strength and muscle mass during resistance training. Despite these potential benefits, no research has supported these claims in human models. Wilborn et al. [103] showed that 8-week supplementation (800 mg of methoxyisoflavone per day) failed to affect body composition or training adaptations, or influence the anabolic/catabolic hormone status or general markers of catabolism in resistance-trained males.

Health Risks

Few considerations about risks related to the intake of sport supplements are needed.

It is self-evident that any medical condition that may contraindicate the use of specific substances must be taken into consideration when deciding to take supplements. Furthermore, athletes and sport practitioners should have clear in mind that dietary supplements should not be used to justify poor food habits. Many athletes, in fact, have a low level of nutritional knowledge and no access to qualified professionals for nutritional counseling. Furthermore, many supplements, such as vitamins and minerals, are considered completely safe being part of the habitual diet, while very high intake for a long time could have negative effects. For example, a Norwegian study reported that high dosages of vitamins C and E [1,000 mg vitamin C and 235 mg of vitamin E (α-tocopherol) per 10 weeks] inhibited the adaptation to strength training in young, healthy volunteers [104].

The daily vitamin and mineral intake through the diet and the amount consumed with common fortified foods, such as cereals, drinks, and yoghurts, should also be taken into consideration. Most public institutions involved in nutrition determined tolerable upper levels or safe upper levels of intake for vitamins and minerals in order to reduce the risk of overconsumption. However, these levels derive generally from few data and lack of consideration about individual variability and sensitivity.

The interaction between supplements is another aspect not always adequately considered; while some compounds work in synergy, others may interact to provide negative outcomes. For all these reasons, caution should be exercised.

In addition, there are also health risks associated with poor manufacturing practice and with the presence of contaminants. Notwithstanding efforts to counteract this problem, some preparations for athletes may be contaminated with harmful or banned substances. To address this concern, the Food and Drug Administration issued rules requiring manufacturers to follow 'current good manufacturing practices' and to ensure that dietary supplements are produced in a 'quality manner, do not contain contaminants or impurities, and are adequately labeled' [105].

Finally, it should be remarked that the effects of supplement use on growth and development of children and adolescents remain unclear, and, thus, the use of supplements by this population should always be discouraged.

Conclusions

In conclusion, nutritional supplements advertised as ergogenic substances are highly accessible and commonly used by athletes at all levels. However, it is extremely important to underline that sport supplements are not for everyone, and oversight of qualified specialists is needed to suggest whether and how to use them. This aspect is particularly critical when considering young athletes who are highly vulnerable to pressures from the media and the prospect of playing sport at increasingly elite levels. Despite the efforts of some scientific and sporting organizations to educate professional as well as amateur athletes about supplement efficacy, safety, and legality, much remains to be done in order to provide as much accurate information as possible. In fact, most of these athletes take supplements and stimulants available online, believing to attenuate fatigue and increase muscle mass and sport performance without knowing the potential health risks of a wrong supplementation. The level of scientific evidence remains the most important approach to identify the effectiveness and safety of each product, and the research has the important role to enforce scientific substantiation proving a cause-effect relationship. Companies should develop scientifically based products by supporting applied research, market the results of studies, and provide dosage instructions for products and other directions for use to help consumers in making informed decisions.

References

1 Kreider RB, Wilborn CD, Taylor L, Campbell B, Almada AL, Collins R, Cooke M, Earnest CP, Greenwood M, Kalman DS, Kerksick CM, Kleiner SM, Leutholtz B, Lopez H, Lowery LM, Mendel R, Smith A, Spano M, Wildman R, Willoughby DS, Ziegenfuss TN, Antonio J: ISSN exercise & sport nutrition review: research & recommendations. J Int Soc Sports Nutr 2010;7:7.

2 Maughan RJ, King DS, Lea T: Dietary supplements. J Sports Sci 2004;22:95–113.

3 McDowall JA: Supplement use by young athletes. J Sports Sci Med 2007;6:337–342.

4 Froiland K, Koszewski W, Hingst J, Kopecky L: Nutritional supplement use among college athletes and their sources of information. Int J Sport Nutr Exerc Metab 2004;14:104–120.

5 http://globenewswire.com/news-release/2015/01/27/700276/10117198/en/Global-Nutrition-and-Supplements-Market-History-Industry-Growth-and-Future-Trends-by-PMR.html (accessed September 18, 2015).

6 www.euromonitor.com/trends-and-developmkent-in-sports-nutrition/report (accessed July 14, 2015).

7 Huang S, Johnson K, Pipe AL: The use of dietary supplements and medications by Canadian athletes at the Atlanta and Sydney Olympic games. Clin J Sports Med 2006;16:27–33.

8 Leone L, Pesce C: Rapporto per l'ISS Istituto Superiore di Sanità. Indagine sul consumo di integratori alimentari e di sostanze illecite per l'aumento delle performance tra utenti delle palestre e sugli effetti di un intervento Informativo. Roma, UISP, CEVAS, 2012.

9 Directive 2002/46/EC of the European Parliament and of the Council of 10 June 2002 on the approximation of the laws of the Member States relating to food supplements. Official J 12.7.2002, L183, pp 51–57.

10 Maughan RJ, Depiesse F, Geyer H: The use of dietary supplements by athletes. J Sports Sci 2007;25(S1): S103–S113.

11 Braun H, Currell K, Stear SJ: Supplements and ergogenic aids; in Susan A: Lanham-New SS, Shirreffs S, Collins A (eds): Sport and Exercise Nutrition. Chichester, Wiley-Blackwell, 2011, vol 9, pp 89–120.

12 EFSA: Scientific Opinion on the substantiation of health claims related to carbohydrate-electrolyte solutions and reduction in rated perceived exertion/effort during exercise (ID 460, 466, 467, 468), enhancement of water absorption during exercise (ID 314, 315, 316, 317, 319, 322, 325, 332, 408, 465, 473, 1168, 1574, 1593, 1618, 4302, 4309), and maintenance of endurance performance (ID 466, 469) pursuant to Article 13(1) of Regulation (EC) No 1924/2006. EFSA J 2011;9:2211.

13 EFSA: Scientific Opinion on the substantiation of a health claim related to glycaemic carbohydrates and recovery of normal muscle function (contraction) after strenuous exercise pursuant to Article 13(5) of Regulation (EC) No 1924/2006. EFSA J 2013;11: 3409.

14 EFSA: Scientific Opinion on the substantiation of health claims related to creatine and increase in physical performance during short-term, high intensity, repeated exercise bouts (ID 739, 1520, 1521, 1522, 1523, 1525, 1526, 1531, 1532, 1533, 1534, 1922, 1923, 1924), increase in endurance capacity (ID 1527, 1535), and increase in endurance performance (ID 1521, 1963) pursuant to Article 13(1) of Regulation (EC) No 1924/2006. EFSA J 2011;9:2303.

15 EFSA: Scientific Opinion on the substantiation of health claims related to vitamin C and protection of DNA, proteins and lipids from oxidative damage (ID 129, 138, 143, 148), antioxidant function of lutein (ID 146), maintenance of vision (ID 141, 142), collagen formation (ID 130, 131, 136, 137, 149), function of the nervous system (ID 133), function of the immune system (ID 134), function of the immune system during and after extreme physical exercise (ID 144), non-haem iron absorption (ID 132, 147), energy-yielding metabolism (ID 135), and relief in case of irritation in the upper respiratory tract (ID 1714, 1715) pursuant to Article 13(1) of Regulation (EC) No 1924/2006. EFSA J 2009;7:1226.

16 EFSA: Scientific Opinion on the substantiation of health claims related to caffeine and increase in physical performance during short-term high-intensity exercise (ID 737, 1486, 1489), increase in endurance performance (ID 737, 1486), increase in endurance capacity (ID 1488) and reduction in the rated perceived exertion/effort during exercise (ID 1488, 1490) pursuant to Article 13(1) of Regulation (EC) No 1924/2006. EFSA J 2011;9:2053.

17 Schubert MM, Astorino TA: A systematic review of the efficacy of ergogenic aids for improving running performance. J Strength Cond Res 2013;27:1699–1707.

18 Evans MW Jr, Ndetan H, Perko M, Williams R, Walker C: Dietary supplement use by children and adolescents in the United States to enhance sport performance. Results of the National Health Interview Survey. J Prim Prev 2012;33:3–12.

19 Engelberg ET, Moston S, Skinner J: Tracking the Development of Attitudes to Doping: A Longitudinal Study of Young Elite Athletes. Report. University of Canberra and Griffith University, 2014, http://www.6minutes.com.au/getmedia/b739564c-a508-402d-98de-9b317d0e17a4/Tracking-the-development-of-attitudes-to-doping-2014-Executive-summary.aspx.

20 Ziegler PJ, Nelson JA, Jonnalagadda SS: Use of dietary supplements by elite figure skaters. Int J Sport Nutr Exerc Metab 2003;13:266–276.

21 Cooper R, Naclerio F, Allgrove J, Jimenez A: Creatine supplementation with specific view to exercise/sports performance: an update. J Int Soc Sports Nutr 2012;9:33.

22 Momaya A, Fawal M, Estes R: Performance-enhancing substances in sports: a review of the literature. Sports Med 2015;45:517–531.

23 Branch JD: Effect of creatine supplementation on body composition and performance: a meta-analysis. Int J Sport Nutr Exerc Metab 2003;13:198–226.

24 Lanhers C, Pereira B, Naughton G, Trousselard M, Lesage FX, Dutheil F: Creatine supplementation and lower limb strength performance: a systematic review and meta-analyses. Sports Med 2015;45:1285–1294.

25 Buford TW, Kreider RB, Stout JR, Greenwood M, Campbell B, Spano M, Ziegenfuss T, Lopez H, Landis J, Antonio J: International Society of Sports Nutrition position stand: creatine supplementation and exercise. J Int Soc Sports Nutr 2007;4:6.

26 Williams J, Abt G, Kilding AE: Effects of creatine monohydrate supplementation on simulated soccer performance. Int J Sports Physiol Perform 2014;9:503–510.

27 da Silveira CL, de Souza TS, Batista GR, de Araújo AT, da Silva JC, de Sousa Mdo S, Marta C, Garrido ND: Is long term creatine and glutamine supplementation effective in enhancing physical performance of military police officers? J Hum Kinet 2014;43:131–138.

28 Kresta JY, Oliver JM, Jagim AR, Fluckey J, Riechman S, Kelly K, Meininger C, Mertens-Talcott SU, Rasmussen C, Kreider RB: Effects of 28 days of beta-alanine and creatine supplementation on muscle carnosine, body composition and exercise performance in recreationally active females. J Int Soc Sports Nutr 2014;11:55.

29 Bassit RA, Pinheiro CH, Vitzel KF, Sproesser AJ, Silveira LR, Curi R: Effect of short-term creatine supplementation on markers of skeletal muscle damage after strenuous contractile activity. Eur J Appl Physiol 2010;108:945–955.

30 Cooke MB, Rybalka E, Williams AD, Cribb PJ, Hayes A: Creatine supplementation enhances muscle force recovery after eccentrically induced muscle damage in healthy individuals. J Int Soc Sports Nutr 2009;6:13.

31 Rahimi R: Creatine supplementation decreases oxidative DNA damage and lipid peroxidation induced by a single bout of resistance exercise. J Strength Cond Res 2011;25:3448–3455.

32 Rucci S, Bonuccelli A, Angelini F, Negro M, Marzatico F: Caffeina: alleata o nemica? SMG 2011;5:40–44, http://www.progettoasco.it/riviste/rivista_simg/2011/05_2011/8.pdf.

33 Committee on Nutrition and the Council on Sports Medicine and Fitness: Clinical report – sports drinks and energy drinks for children and adolescents: are they appropriate? Pediatrics 2011;127:1182–1189.

34 Bishop D: Dietary supplements and team-sport performance. Sports Med 2010;40:995–1017.

35 Ganio MS, Klau JF, Casa DJ, Armstrong LE, Maresh CM: Effect of caffeine on sport-specific endurance performance: a systematic review. J Strength Cond Res 2009;23:315–324.
36 Goldstein ER, Ziegenfuss T, Kalman D, Kreider R, Campbell B, Wilborn C, Taylor L, Willoughby D, Stout J, Graves BS, Wildman R, Ivy JL, Spano M, Smith AE, Antonio J: International Society of Sports Nutrition position stand: caffeine and performance. J Int Soc Sports Nutr 2010;7:5.
37 Shearer J, Graham TE: Performance effects and metabolic consequences of caffeine and caffeinated energy drink consumption on glucose disposal. Nutr Rev 2014;72(suppl 1):121–136.
38 Seifert SM, Schaechter JL, Hershorin ER, Lipshultz SE: Health effects of energy drinks on children, adolescents, and young adults. Pediatrics 2011;127:511–528.
39 Abian P, Del Coso J, Salinero JJ, Gallo-Salazar C, Areces F, Ruiz-Vicente D, Lara B, Soriano L, Muñoz V, Abian-Vicen J: The ingestion of a caffeinated energy drink improves jump performance and activity patterns in elite badminton players. J Sports Sci 2015;33:1042–1050.
40 Del Coso J, Portillo J, Salinero JJ, Lara B, Abian-Vicen J, Areces F: Caffeinated energy drinks improve high-speed running in elite field hockey players. Int J Sport Nutr Exerc Metab 2016;26:26–32.
41 Abian-Vicen J, Puente C, Salinero JJ, González-Millán C, Areces F, Muñoz G, Muñoz-Guerra J, Del Coso J: A caffeinated energy drink improves jump performance in adolescent basketball players. Amino Acids 2014;46:1333–1341.
42 Lara B, Gonzalez-Millán C, Salinero JJ, Abian-Vicen J, Areces F, Barbero-Alvarez JC, Muñoz V, Portillo LJ, Gonzalez-Rave JM, Del Coso J: Caffeine-containing energy drink improves physical performance in female soccer players. Amino Acids 2014;46:1385–1392.
43 Del Coso J, Ramírez JA, Muñoz G, Portillo J, Gonzalez-Millán C, Muñoz V, Barbero-Álvarez JC, Muñoz-Guerra J: Caffeine-containing energy drink improves physical performance of elite rugby players during a simulated match. Appl Physiol Nutr Metab 2013;38:368–374.
44 Del Coso J, Muñoz-Fernández VE, Muñoz G, Fernández-Elías VE, Ortega JF, Hamouti N, Barbero JC, Muñoz-Guerra J: Effects of a caffeine-containing energy drink on simulated soccer performance. PLoS One 2012;7:e31380.
45 Campbell B, Wilborn C, La Bounty P, Taylor L, Nelson MT, Greenwood M, Ziegenfuss TN, Lopez HL, Hoffman JR, Stout JR, Schmitz S, Collins R, Kalman DS, Antonio J, Kreider RB: International Society of Sports Nutrition position stand: energy drinks. J Int Soc Sports Nutr 2013;10:1.
46 Gallo-Salazar C, Areces F, Abián-Vicén J, Lara B, Salinero JJ, Gonzalez-Millán C, Portillo J, Muñoz V, Juarez D, Del Coso J: Enhancing physical performance in elite junior tennis players with a caffeinated energy drink. Int J Sports Physiol Perform 2015;10:305–310.
47 Wilson JM, Fitschen PJ, Campbell B, Wilson GJ, Zanchi N, Taylor L, Wilborn C, Kalman DS, Stout JR, Hoffman JR, Ziegenfuss TN, Lopez HL, Kreider RB, Smith-Ryan AE, Antonio J: International Society of Sports Nutrition position stand: beta-hydroxy-beta-methylbutyrate (HMB). J Int Soc Sports Nutr 2013;10:6.
48 Zanchi NE, Gerlinger-Romero F, Guimarães-Ferreira L, de Siqueira Filho MA, Felitti V, Lira FS, Seelaender M, Lancha AH Jr: HMB supplementation: clinical and athletic performance-related effects and mechanisms of action. Amino Acids 2011;40:1015–1025.
49 Wilson GJ, Wilson JM, Manninen AH: Effects of beta-hydroxy-beta-methylbutyrate (HMB) on exercise performance and body composition across varying levels of age, sex, and training experience: a review. Nutr Metab (Lond) 2008;5:1.
50 Jówko E, Ostaszewski P, Jank M, Sacharuk J, Zieniewicz A, Wilczak J, Nissen S: Creatine and beta-hydroxy-beta-methylbutyrate (HMB) additively increase lean body mass and muscle strength during a weight-training program. Nutrition 2001;17:558–666.
51 Knitter AE, Panton L, Rathmacher JA, Petersen A, Sharp R: Effects of beta-hydroxy-beta-methylbutyrate on muscle damage after a prolonged run. J Appl Physiol (1985) 2000;89:1340–1344.
52 Gallagher PM, Carrithers JA, Godard MP, Schulze KE, Trappe SW: Beta-hydroxy-beta-methylbutyrate ingestion. Part I: effects on strength and fat free mass. Med Sci Sports Exerc 2000;32:2109–2115.
53 Nissen S, Sharp R, Ray M, Rathmacher JA, Rice D, Fuller JC Jr, Connelly AS, Abumrad N: Effect of leucine metabolite beta-hydroxy-beta-methylbutyrate on muscle metabolism during resistance-exercise training. J Appl Physiol (1985) 1996;81:2095–2104.
54 Kraemer WJ, Hatfield DL, Volek JS, Fragala MS, Vingren JL, Anderson JM, Spiering BA, Thomas GA, Ho JY, Quann EE, Izquierdo M, Häkkinen K, Maresh CM: Effects of amino acids supplement on physiological adaptations to resistance training. Med Sci Sports Exerc 2009;41:1111–1121.
55 Vukovich MD, Dreifort GD: Effect of beta-hydroxy beta-methylbutyrate on the onset of blood lactate accumulation and V(O)(2) peak in endurance-trained cyclists. J Strength Cond Res 2001;15:491–497.
56 Molfino A, Gioia G, Rossi Fanelli F, Muscaritoli M: Beta-hydroxy-beta-methylbutyrate supplementation in health and disease: a systematic review of randomized trials. Amino Acids 2013;45:1273–1292.

57 Portal S, Eliakim A, Nemet D, Halevy O, Zadik Z: Effect of HMB supplementation on body composition, fitness, hormonal profile and muscle damage indices. J Pediatr Endocrinol Metab 2010;23:641–650.
58 Rowlands DS, Thomson JS: Effects of beta-hydroxy-beta-methylbutyrate supplementation during resistance training on strength, body composition, and muscle damage in trained and untrained young men: a meta-analysis. J Strength Cond Res 2009;23:836–846.
59 Palisin T, Stacy JJ: Beta-hydroxy-beta-methylbutyrate and its use in athletics. Curr Sports Med Rep 2005;4:220–223.
60 EFSA: Scientific Opinion on the substantiation of health claims related to β-hydroxy β-methylbutyrate monohydrate (HMB) alone or in combination with α-ketoisocaproic acid (KIC) and reduction of muscle tissue damage during exercise (ID 1577, 1584), increase in lean body mass (ID 1579, 1582, 1583), increase in muscle strength (ID 1578, 1583, 1587), increase in endurance performance (ID 1580, 1581), skeletal muscle tissue repair (ID 1586) and faster recovery from muscle fatigue after exercise (ID 1576, 1585) pursuant to Article 13(1) of Regulation (EC) No 1924/2006. EFSA J 2011;9:2227.
61 Yavari A, Javadi M, Mirmiran P, Bahadoran Z: Exercise-induced oxidative stress and dietary antioxidants. Asian J Sports Med 2015;6:e24898.
62 Brisswalter J, Louis J: Vitamin supplementation benefits in master athletes. Sports Med 2014;44:311–318.
63 Braakhuis AJ: Effect of vitamin C supplements on physical performance. Curr Sports Med Rep 2012; 11:180–184.
64 Lukaski HC: Vitamin and mineral status: effects on physical performance. Nutrition 2004;20:632–644.
65 Theodorou AA, Nikolaidis MG, Paschalis V, Koutsias S, Panayiotou G, Fatouros IG, Koutedakis Y, Jamurtas AZ: No effect of antioxidant supplementation on muscle performance and blood redox status adaptations to eccentric training. Am J Clin Nutr 2011;93:1373–1383.
66 Yfanti C, Akerström T, Nielsen S, Nielsen AR, Mounier R, Mortensen OH, Lykkesfeldt J, Rose AJ, Fischer CP, Pedersen BK: Antioxidant supplementation does not alter endurance training adaptation. Med Sci Sports Exerc 2010;42:1388–1395.
67 Zoppi CC, Hohl R, Silva FC, Lazarim FL, Neto JM, Stancanneli M, Macedo DV: Vitamin C and E supplementation effects in professional soccer players under regular training. J Int Soc Sports Nutr 2006;3: 37–44.
68 Braakhuis AJ, Hopkins WG: Impact of dietary antioxidants on sport performance: a review. Sports Med 2015;45:939–955.
69 Romano-Ely BC, Todd MK, Saunders MJ, Laurent TS: Effect of an isocaloric carbohydrate-protein-antioxidant drink on cycling performance. Med Sci Sports Exerc 2006;38:1608–1616.
70 Kobayashi Y: Effect of Vitamin E on Aerobic Work Performance in Man during Exposure to Hypoxic Hypoxia; dissertation. Albuquerque, University of New Mexico, 1974.
71 Simon-Schnass I, Pabst H: Influence of vitamin E on physical performance. Int J Vitam Nutr Res 1988;58: 49–54.
72 Medved I, Brown MJ, Bjorksten AR, Murphy KT, Petersen AC, Sostaric S, Gong X, McKenna MJ: N-acetylcysteine enhances muscle cysteine and glutathione availability and attenuates fatigue during prolonged exercise in endurance-trained individuals. J Appl Physiol (1985) 2004;97:1477–1485.
73 McKenna MJ, Medved I, Goodman CA, Brown MJ, Bjorksten AR, Murphy KT, Petersen AC, Sostaric S, Gong X: N-acetylcysteine attenuates the decline in muscle Na^+, K^+-pump activity and delays fatigue during prolonged exercise in humans. J Physiol 2006;576:279–288.
74 Huupponen MR, Mäkinen LH, Hyvönen PM, Sen CK, Rankinen T, Väisänen S, Rauramaa R: The effect of N-acetylcysteine on exercise-induced priming of human neutrophils. A chemiluminescence study. Int J Sports Med 1995;16:399–403.
75 Slattery KM, Dascombe B, Wallace LK, Bentley DJ, Coutts AJ: Effect of N-acetylcysteine on cycling performance after intensified training. Med Sci Sports Exerc 2014;46:1114–1123.
76 Trewin AJ, Petersen AC, Billaut F, McQuade LR, McInerney BV, Stepto NK: N-acetylcysteine alters substrate metabolism during high-intensity cycle exercise in well-trained humans. Appl Physiol Nutr Metab 2013;38:1217–1227.
77 Petersen AC, McKenna MJ, Medved I, Murphy KT, Brown MJ, Della Gatta P, Cameron-Smith D: Infusion with the antioxidant N-acetylcysteine attenuates early adaptive responses to exercise in human skeletal muscle. Acta Physiol (Oxf) 2012;204:382–392.
78 Díaz-Castro J, Guisado R, Kajarabille N, García C, Guisado IM, de Teresa C, Ochoa JJ: Coenzyme Q(10) supplementation ameliorates inflammatory signaling and oxidative stress associated with strenuous exercise. Eur J Nutr 2012;51:791–799.
79 Leelarungrayub D, Sawattikanon N, Klaphajone J, Pothongsunan P, Bloomer RJ: Coenzyme Q10 supplementation decreases oxidative stress and improves physical performance in young swimmers: a pilot study. Open Sports Med J 2010;4:1–8.

80 Zeppilli P, Merlino B, De Luca A, Palmeri V, Sanitini C, Vannicelli R, La Rosa Gangi M, Caccese R, Cameli S, Servidei S, Ricci E, Silvestri G, Lippa S, Oradei A, Littaru P: Influence of coenzyme-Q10 on physical work capacity in athletes, sedentary people and patients with mitochondrial disease; in Folkers K, Littaru GP, Yamagami T (eds): Biomedical and Clinical Aspects of Coenzyme Q. Amsterdam, Elsevier, 1991, vol 6, pp 541–545.
81 Cerioli G, Tirelli F, Mustani L: Effect of CoQ10 on the metabolic response to work; in Folkers K, Littaru GP, Yamagami T (eds): Biomedical and Clinical Aspects of Coenzyme Q. Amsterdam, Elsevier, 1991, vol 6, pp 521–524.
82 Powers SK, DeRuisseau KC, Quindry J, Hamilton KL: Dietary antioxidants and exercise. J Sports Sci 2004;22:81–94.
83 EFSA: Scientific Opinion on the substantiation of health claims related to coenzyme Q10 and contribution to normal energy-yielding metabolism (ID 1508, 1512, 1720, 1912, 4668), maintenance of normal blood pressure (ID 1509, 1721, 1911), protection of DNA, proteins and lipids from oxidative damage (ID 1510), contribution to normal cognitive function (ID 1511), maintenance of normal blood cholesterol concentrations (ID 1721) and increase in endurance capacity and/or endurance performance (ID 1913) pursuant to Article 13(1) of Regulation (EC) No 1924/20061. EFSA J 2010;8:1793.
84 Shay KP, Moreau RF, Smith EJ, Smith AR, Hagen TM: Alpha-lipoic acid as a dietary supplement: molecular mechanisms and therapeutic potential. Biochim Biophys Acta 2009;1790:1149–1160.
85 Morawin B, Turowski D, Naczk M, Siatkowski I, Zembron-Lacny A: The combination of α-lipoic acid intake with eccentric exercise modulates erythropoietin release. Biol Sport 2014;31:179–185.
86 Zembron-Lacny A, Slowinska-Lisowska M, Szygula Z, Witkowski K, Stefaniak T, Dziubek W: Assessment of the antioxidant effectiveness of alpha-lipoic acid in healthy men exposed to muscle-damaging exercise. J Physiol Pharmacol 2009;60:139–143.
87 Santhakumar AB, Bulmer AC, Singh I: A review of the mechanisms and effectiveness of dietary polyphenols in reducing oxidative stress and thrombotic risk. J Hum Nutr Diet 2014;27:1–21.
88 Del Bo' C, Porrini M, Fracassetti D, Campolo J, Klimis-Zacas D, Riso P: A single serving of blueberry *(V. corymbosum)* modulates peripheral arterial dysfunction induced by acute cigarette smoking in young volunteers: a randomized-controlled trial. Food Funct 2014;5:3107–3116.
89 Riso P, Klimis-Zacas D, Del Bo' C, Martini D, Campolo J, Vendrame S, Møller P, Loft S, De Maria R, Porrini M: Effect of a wild blueberry *(Vaccinium angustifolium)* drink intervention on markers of oxidative stress, inflammation and endothelial function in humans with cardiovascular risk factors. Eur J Nutr 2013;52:949–961.
90 Del Bo' C, Riso P, Campolo J, Møller P, Loft S, Klimis-Zacas D, Brambilla A, Rizzolo A, Porrini M: A single portion of blueberry (*Vaccinium corymbosum* L) improves protection against DNA damage but not vascular function in healthy male volunteers. Nutr Res 2013;33:220–227.
91 Chang WH, Hu SP, Huang YF, Yeh TS, Liu JF: Effect of purple sweet potato leaves consumption on exercise-induced oxidative stress and IL-6 and HSP72 levels. J Appl Physiol (1985) 2010;109:1710–1715.
92 McAnulty SR, McAnulty LS, Nieman DC, Dumke CL, Morrow JD, Utter AC, Henson DA, Proulx WR, George GL: Consumption of blueberry polyphenols reduces exercise-induced oxidative stress compared to vitamin C. Nutr Res 2004;24:209–221.
93 Lafay S, Jan C, Nardon K, Lemaire B, Ibarra A, Roller M, Houvenaeghel M, Juhel C, Cara L: Grape extract improves antioxidant status and physical performance in elite male athletes. J Sports Sci Med 2009;8:468–480.
94 Kressler J, Millard-Stafford M, Warren GL: Quercetin and endurance exercise capacity: a systematic review and meta-analysis. Med Sci Sports Exerc 2011; 43:2396–2404.
95 Yarahmadi M, Askari G, Kargarfard M, Ghiasvand R, Hoseini M, Mohamadi H, Asadi A: The effect of anthocyanin supplementation on body composition, exercise performance and muscle damage indices in athletes. Int J Prev Med 2014;5:1594–1600.
96 Pilaczynska-Szczesniak L, Skarpanska-Steinborn A, Deskur E, Basta P, Horoszkiewicz-Hassan M: The influence of chokeberry juice supplementation on the reduction of oxidative stress resulting from an incremental rowing ergometer exercise. Int J Sport Nutr Exerc Metab 2005;15:48–58.
97 Bowtell JL, Sumners DP, Dyer A, Fox P, Mileva KN: Montmorency cherry juice reduces muscle damage caused by intensive strength exercise. Med Sci Sports Exerc 2011;43:1544–1551.
98 Trombold JR, Reinfeld AS, Casler JR, Coyle EF: The effect of pomegranate juice supplementation on strength and soreness after eccentric exercise. J Strength Cond Res 2011;25:1782–1788.
99 Rennie MJ, Ahmed A, Khogali SE, Low SY, Hundal HS, Taylor PM: Glutamine metabolism and transport in skeletal muscle and heart and their clinical relevance. J Nutr 1996;126:1142S–1149S.

100 Varnier M, Leese GP, Thompson J, Rennie MJ: Stimulatory effect of glutamine on glycogen accumulation in human skeletal muscle. Am J Physiol 1995;269:E309–E315.

101 EFSA: Scientific Opinion on the substantiation of health claims related to L-glutamine and growth or maintenance of muscle mass (ID 719, 722, 3185), faster restoration of muscle glycogen stores after strenuous exercise (ID 434, 699, 701, 723, 1569), skeletal muscle tissue repair (ID 721), maintenance of normal neurological function (ID 662, 700), increased attention (ID 700, 1570), improvement of working memory (ID 700, 1570), maintenance of defence against pathogenic gastro-intestinal microorganisms (ID 452), gut protein synthesis (ID 701), decreasing gut permeability (ID 701), and stimulating immunological responses (ID 1568) pursuant to Article 13(1) of Regulation (EC) No 1924/20061. EFSA J 2011;9:2225.

102 Wei P, Liu M, Chen Y, Chen DC: Systematic review of soy isoflavone supplements on osteoporosis in women. Asian Pac J Trop Med 2012;5:243–248.

103 Wilborn CD, Taylor LW, Campbell BI, Kerksick C, Rasmussen CJ, Greenwood M, Kreider RB: Effects of methoxyisoflavone, ecdysterone, and sulfo-polysaccharide supplementation on training adaptations in resistance-trained males. J Int Soc Sports Nutr 2006;3:19–27.

104 Paulsen G, Hamarsland H, Cumming KT, Johansen RE, Hulmi JJ, Børsheim E, Wiig H, Garthe I, Raastad T: Vitamin C and E supplementation alters protein signalling after a strength training session, but not muscle growth during 10 weeks of training. J Physiol 2014;592:5391–5408.

105 Overview of the Implementation of the Current Good Manufacturing Practices for Dietary Supplements Guidance for Industry. http://www.fda.gov/Food/GuidanceRegulation/CGMP/ucm173996.htm.

Marisa Porrini
Division of Human Nutrition, Department of Food,
Environmental and Nutritional Sciences, Università degli Studi di Milano
Via G. Celoria 2, IT–20133 Milan (Italy)
E-Mail marisa.porrini@unimi.it

Use of Performance-Enhancing Endocrine Drugs (Doping) in Competitive and Recreational Sports Activity

Lanfranco F, Strasburger CJ (eds): Sports Endocrinology.
Front Horm Res. Basel, Karger, 2016, vol 47, pp 153–167 (DOI: 10.1159/000445177)

Methods for Doping Detection

Federico Ponzetto[a] · Sylvain Giraud[a] · Nicolas Leuenberger[a] · Julien Boccard[b] · Raul Nicoli[a] · Norbert Baume[a] · Serge Rudaz[b] · Martial Saugy[a]

[a]Swiss Laboratory for Doping Analyses, Epalinges, and University Center of Legal Medicine Geneva and Lausanne, Centre Hospitalier Universitaire Vaudois and University of Lausanne, Lausanne, and [b]Laboratory of Pharmaceutical Analytical Chemistry, School of Pharmaceutical Sciences, University of Geneva, Geneva, Switzerland

Abstract

Over the past few years, the World Anti-Doping Agency (WADA) has focused its efforts on detecting not only small prohibited molecules, but also larger endogenous molecules such as hormones, in the view of implementing an endocrinological module in the Athlete Biological Passport (ABP). In this chapter, the detection of two major types of hormones used for doping, growth hormone (GH) and endogenous anabolic androgenic steroids (EAASs), will be discussed: a brief historical background followed by a description of state-of-the-art methods applied by accredited anti-doping laboratories will be provided and then current research trends outlined. In addition, microRNAs (miRNAs) will also be presented as a new class of biomarkers for doping detection.

Growth Hormone

The ergogenic effects of GH and related risks, as well as potential methods for detecting its abuse for anti-doping purposes, have been reviewed by multiple authors. In this context, it is important to note that short-term administration of GH does not increase exercise capacity. A review by Erotokritou-Mulligan et al. [1], published in 2001, addresses all of these topics. Since at least 1996, it has been recognized that multiple tests are required to detect GH abuse; therefore, a ratio or formula combining different values must be used for this purpose [2].

The GH-2000 Study Group published the results of a 4-week GH administration study demonstrating that multiple markers are significantly altered following GH administration, some of which can be used to detect GH abuse [3]. The same markers were also tested in the context of exercise, because their usefulness would be drastically curtailed if their levels were also significantly modified by strenuous exercise. Wallace et al. [4] performed a study in trained adults showing that exercise did indeed induce changes in some of these markers, but that these changes were smaller than those resulting from GH abuse. This promising approach was set aside, however, due to the limited availability of the required tests. Attention was instead directed toward another test based on the concentrations of different isoforms of endogenously produced GH. Most endogenous GH is produced by the pituitary gland as a 22-kDa protein, but an important part of this pituitary GH suffers from errors during the translation between DNA and protein that results in 20- or 17-kDa GH isoforms. The isoform-based approach is based on the measurement of the relative concentrations of these isoforms. Because GH is autoregulated by its own serum concentration, the presence of recombinant GH should attenuate the endogenous production of GH. Consequently, in the presence of recombinant GH, the 22-kDa isoform (the only one produced by the pharmaceutical industry) will be abundant, whereas the other isoforms will be scarce or absent. The published approach uses a ratio of two different ELISAs that measure GH isoform concentrations in different ways. The ratio allows us to ignore large changes in GH concentration and is thus very robust [5]. However, while this approach is robust from a physiological point of view, it suffers from a major bias, i.e. a short detection window. This means that if an athlete abuses GH, but does not provide blood to the anti-doping authorities within 48 h after GH intake, he should not fear detection.

In 2007, the use of markers induced by GH abuse was validated, resulting in the GH-2000 Score (in the following referred to as Score) calculated according to a formula that takes age into account, the most preeminent confounding factor [6]. Unfortunately, data were not available regarding other factors that might influence the Score. Because the isoform approach is more suitable for detecting recombinant human GH abuse, the simple ratio described above was sufficiently robust to normalize age, sport, ethnicity, and other potential confounding factors. The only potential risk was the aforementioned possibility of effort-induced changes; nonetheless, the test was implemented after taking precautions described in the anti-doping blood collection protocol. A full validation study was published [7], and the first cases appeared at the end of 2010. This method could yet be improved, in order to increase the detection window, using the same basic approach, e.g. by developing tests based on antibodies that are both very specific for individual isoforms and sensitive enough to measure infinitesimal quantities of each isoform [8].

After numerous studies and publications, the Holt group was able to provide sufficient documentation to convince WADA of the credibility and robustness of the GH marker approach. They showed that reanalytical and sample storage conditions did not change the Score by more than 0.5 units, and that no significant differences could be detected between the various tested conditions. The situation was almost identical with regard to ethnic variations or the young (minor) athletes. The Scores were all within the reference population values, allowing the decision limit (DL) to be established, accepted, and published in advance of the 2012 Olympic Games in London. Some issues persisted regarding plasma volume variation related to hydration, but the range of such changes was small compared to the DL and mean Score [9]. After inclusion of more results, the final DLs were published, and the test was implemented in anti-doping laboratories [10].

Currently, there are two ways to detect GH abuse, both of which are based on changes in GH-related pathways. Neither of these approaches involves direct identification of recombinant GH. Indeed, direct detection of recombinant growth factors is difficult due to the endogenous origin of these factors and their very low concentrations. Liquid chromatography (LC) mass spectrometry (MS) could be used, but it requires concentrations higher than the physiological range or preliminary concentration of GH.

The biological passport represents a powerful tool for improving the global efficiency of the anti-doping system, and detection of GH abuse would fit perfectly into longitudinal follow-up because markers constitute the foundation of the ABP. For now, however, follow-up based on both isoforms and markers would be very expensive, and there is no guarantee that it would be significantly more informative than either test taken alone. The sensitivity and specificity of the GH longitudinal follow-up must be improved before it can be used for anti-doping purposes. For example, specificity could be increased using markers related to disease, injuries, or other confounding factors.

A major study was conducted during the Athletic World Championship held in 2011 in Daegu, Korea. The results obtained by Robinson et al. [11] from these samples indicated that the Score is related to the type of exercise performed by the athlete. However, because the tools used for this study were those described for the London Olympics, which are no longer used as a reference for WADA, it was not possible to determine whether this difference was related to a difference in the prevalence of doping between the two populations of athletes or to physiological changes in the growth markers. Figure 1 presents a multivariate analysis performed on these results. For each plot, the results were normalized to remove all influencing factors except the factor under study. The difference between men and women was tested, as was the influence of discipline. For this purpose, a threshold value of 3 min of effort was set with the aim of discriminating between endurance and nonendurance disciplines. According to this limit, the 3,000-meter steeplechase was defined as the shortest endurance discipline. Normally, the age of the athlete is included as a correction factor in such formulas, so this normalization was also performed. Other factors that are not displayed (because they do not exert any significant influence) were blood collection time, intense training within 2 h before collection, and time at elevations

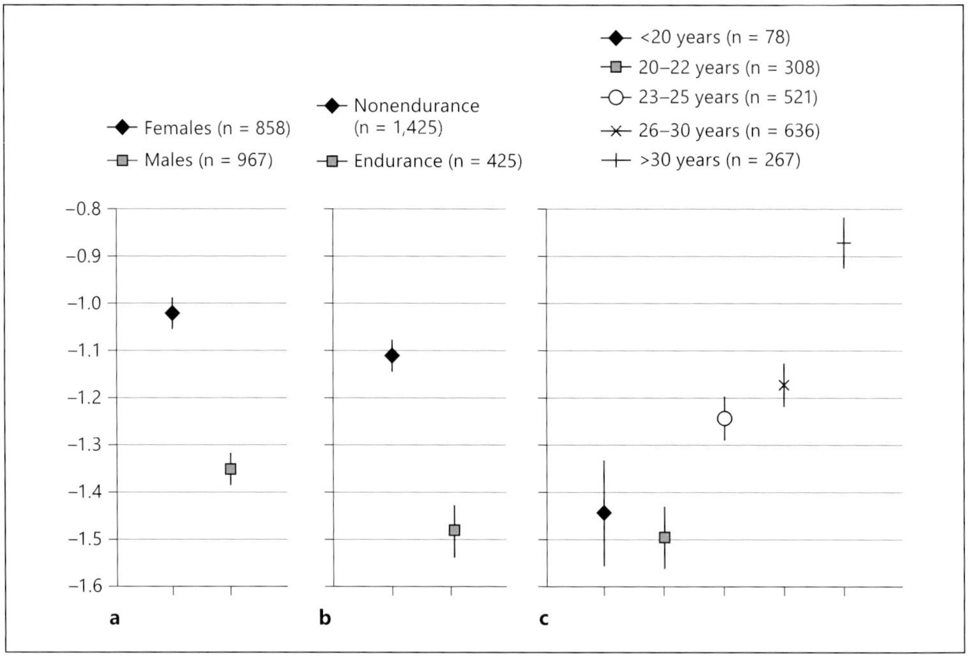

Fig. 1. Plot of multivariate analyses. For each influencing factor, the Score from all samples was corrected to remove the influence of the others factors. The plots present means ± SD of the Score distribution based on main factors: gender of the samples (**a**), type of discipline (endurance: from a 3,000-meter run, nonendurance: shorter event; **b**), and age of the athletes (**c**).

greater than 1,000 m. Importantly, the measurement uncertainty of the Score was 0.5 units. Therefore, a difference smaller than 0.5 units, even if significant from a mathematical point of view, should be considered to reflect the normal variation in the analytical method.

In the same population, the same analysis was performed on results obtained using the isoform approach. As common in anti-doping, 2 tests must be used to confirm abnormal results: screening and confirmation. These two tests for the isoform approach are referred to as kit 1 and kit 2. Both can be used for any step, but both must present abnormal results to open a 'doping case'. For kit 1, no parameter (including gender) caused any significant difference. By contrast, for kit 2, gender slightly influenced the ratio. For the results from this kit, training performed within 2 h before collection was significant. The means ± SD were 0.49 ± 0.03 and 0.56 ± 0.01 for subjects who did or did not engage in training, respectively. Once again, the difference (0.07) has no practical importance because it is smaller than the method uncertainty.

These Daegu samples were used to determine the current DL for the marker approach using the most up-to-date approved tools and tests. Analysis of the data revealed variations in mean Scores among different disciplines. Even if these observed alterations were small from a practical standpoint, they could be related to two main root causes: physiological changes induced by discipline or higher doping prevalence in certain disciplines. In the first case, the influence of the discipline should be included in the interpretation of the results, e.g. as a note given to the management authorities along with the report indicating the presence of growth factor abuse. In the second case, the test demonstrates its ability to detect small changes due to doping, and also indicates that the current DLs are too high because they would include cheating athletes.

In summary, Score variations can be linked to athlete physiologies, to doping prevalence, and to intra-individual factors. The first situation indicates reduced specificity, whereas the second indicates reduced sensitivity, and the third situation is the root of the Score distribution. In any case, some care should be taken when interpreting the results.

Endogenous Anabolic Androgenic Steroids

Steroid Profile

Screening and quantification of EAASs in urine matrix are part of the routine analytical menu proposed by WADA-accredited laboratories. EAASs constitute the so-called urinary steroid profile, which encompasses the concentrations of the free and glucuro-conjugated fractions of the main natural anabolic and androgenic hormone testosterone (T) and its epimer, epitestosterone (E), as well as the four main T metabolites [androsterone (A), etiocholanolone (Etio), 5α-androstane-3α, 17β-diol (5α-Adiol), and 5β-androstane-3α,17β-diol (5β-Adiol)] and ratios such as T/E, A/Etio, 5α-Adiol/5β-Adiol, and A/T. This steroid profile has been used since a paper by Donike [12], published in the early 1990s, provided proof of principle for steroid profile evaluation as a method for detecting T misuse. Since then, the rules for interpreting the natural or abnormal variability of measured biomarkers have changed over time. Although the T/E ratio is stable within an individual, it is also the parameter most strongly influenced following exogenous input of T or similar compounds. In 1983, an initial T/E population limit of 6 was established, above which an athlete would be suspected of T abuse. This population-based threshold was then adjusted to 4 in 2004 when WADA issued the first version of the technical document describing the reporting and evaluation guidance for T, E, other endogenous steroids, and the T/E ratio [13]. In the same document, WADA provided specific instructions for performing additional analyses using gas chromatography-combustion-isotope ratio MS (GC-C-IRMS) on samples exhibiting suspicious concentrations of steroid biomarkers. GC-C-IRMS is an effective analytical tool that allows to determine the source of the investigated compounds, such as T, based on variations in stable isotopes such as ^{12}C and ^{13}C. Measurement of the carbon isotopic ratio provides data that can be used to determine whether T and related compounds are endogenously produced or exogenously administered. Between 2004 and 2014, additional analyses using GC-C-IRMS technology were performed on samples with EAAS concentrations above the thresholds specified in the WADA technical document (i.e. T or E >200 ng/ml, A or Etio >10,000 ng/ml, and dehydroepiandrosterone >100 ng/ml) [13].

Since 2014, the population-based approach to the interpretation of steroid profiles was replaced by the adaptive model integrated in the steroidal module of the ABP. This statistical methodology was adapted from the hematological module of the same ABP that has been in force since 2008; its objective is to focus on specific quantifiable biomarkers and follow them over time for each individual athlete. At the beginning of longitudinal follow-up, population reference limits are considered in order to confirm that markers fall within the normal range; as the amount of data increases for a given athlete, the limits are continually adjusted according to the individual variability in the investigated parameters (fig. 2). Consequently, the ABP is based on an adaptive model derived from Bayesian statistics that integrates heterogeneous and confounding factors to reveal the effects of doping behaviors or pathologies that could impact the measured biomarkers.

Although the preanalytical and analytical conditions are well defined for the blood parameters measured in the hematological module of the ABP, the quantification of EAASs in urine suffers from greater inconsistencies due to confounding factors highlighted in several published papers [14] and in the latest version of the WADA technical document *Endogenous Anabolic Androgenic Steroids: Measurement and Reporting*, compiled when the steroidal module was launched in 2014 and revised in 2016 [15]. The main factors influencing urinary measurements of the steroid profile were classified as endogenous or exogenous. Endogenous factors include the athlete's gender, age, and ethnicity, but also genetic polymorphisms linked to androgen metabolism; together, they set the baseline for an individual but also contribute to the 'natural' variation in the profile over long periods of time. On the other hand, exogenous factors such as drugs, medications, and diet are acknowledged as sources of variation in steroid metabolism and excretion from the body. Bacterial contamination has also an important influence on measured steroid concentrations in urine matrix.

Considering all the technical issues regarding EAAS quantification in urine and the high level of expertise needed to rationally evaluate an individual passport, the ABP steroidal module must evolve to increase its specificity and selectivity for use in the fight against doping. The ABP modules are not only useful for deterring doping with T and related compounds, or by blood manipulation, but are also widely used by anti-doping organizations to select and target suspicious athletes for more intensive testing.

Steroidomic Approach

The steroidal module of the ABP clearly improved our ability to detect EAAS misuse; however, this approach is still limited to monitoring of well-known and established compounds, and its performance remains somewhat limited by the choice of param-

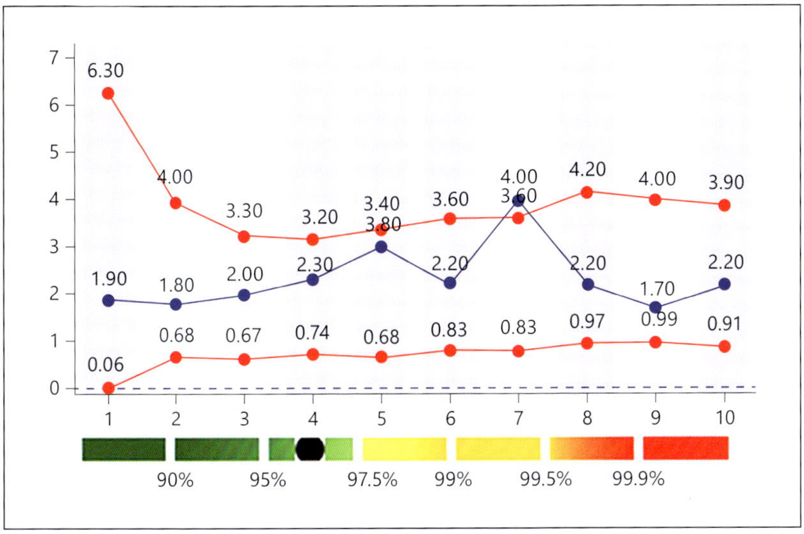

Fig. 2. Longitudinal monitoring of T/E, as implemented in the ABP.

eters that are introduced in the Bayesian adaptive model. Therefore, doping control might still greatly benefit from the addition of relevant parameters to the ABP, including new steroid biomarkers. In this context, the recent profusion of information provided by holistic approaches ('omics') has facilitated innovation. Indeed, metabolomics in general and steroidomics in particular open the door to simultaneous untargeted evaluation of a large number of compounds, and thus represent promising strategies for monitoring of changes in the levels and ratios of endogenous steroids.

Because steroid metabolites have a wide variety of physicochemical properties and concentration levels, ranging from picomolar to millimolar, major efforts are needed to provide analytical tools that can detect, quantify, or identify large numbers of compounds in single analyses of complex samples. One analytical platform particularly suitable for such purposes is the combination of ultrahigh-pressure LC (UHPLC) with high-resolution MS. High-resolution MS devices, especially time-of-flight (TOF), tandem quadrupole (QTOF), and Orbitrap-based instruments, have the ability to acquire data over a wide range of masses (e.g. *m/z* 95–1,000) with a broad dynamic range, highly accurate measurement of mass, and high sensitivity. Modern TOF/MS and tandem QTOF/MS instruments have performances comparable to that of the Orbitrap, but faster acquisition speeds (up to 100 Hz) [16]. However, in contrast to Orbitrap technology, working at very high resolution (up to 80,000 full width at half maximum) impacts detection sensitivity. One advantage of Orbitrap-based instruments is the availability of polarity switching, which allows analysis of both acidic and basic analytes within the same run, whereas with most TOF-based devices two independent injections are required. Therefore, high-resolution MS instruments can ionize and detect thousands of compounds within a single experiment, making them perfectly suitable not only for screening methods but also for untargeted data acquisition, raising the possibility for retrospective examination of raw data without additional analyses [17].

Jeanneret et al. [18] proposed a workflow (fig. 3) for steroidomic analysis. The first step in this scheme is untargeted MS acquisition that can be performed in a generic way, with complementary determinations performed on the same sample (e.g. different ionization processes, sample preparation procedures, or LC stationary phases). Each of these experiments generates large amounts of data containing many thousands of peaks, which can be summarized in a list of features defined by an *m/z* value eluting at a given retention time (t_R) with an associated intensity (m/z@t_R@intensity); furthermore, a single analyte may correspond to several features, such as isotopic peaks, adducts, or in-source fragments. Hence, after acquisition, the grouping of ions belonging to the same molecule (ion annotation) must be performed. Because the inclusion of nonpertinent features can dramatically affect processing speed and data interpretation, another crucial processing step is data denoising. Once properly annotated features are obtained, the next step consists in the signal separation of the 'steroidome' from the metabolome in the acquired data. For this purpose, the use of a steroid database gathering entries from steroids comprised in the Human Metabolome Database or LIPID MASS combined with empirical data including exact mass, MS, MS/MS spectra, and t_R should serve as a basis for (1) filtering features and reducing the initial data dimensionality (leading to easier statistical and biological interpretations), and (2) biomarker identification. The final step of this workflow, which represents the bottleneck of this class of approach, is feature identification. Different levels of identification can be achieved, as summarized by Dunn et al. [19]:

- *level 1:* features matching a steroid already identified using an authentic chemical standard by comparison of exact mass, MS/MS, and t_R;
- *level 2:* features matching steroids with the same exact mass and MS/MS spectra, and
- *level 3:* features matching steroids with the same exact mass.

Because authentic standards are sometimes unavailable for steroids and their metabolites, prior time-consuming syntheses, or other identification strategies, a further reduction in relevant features must be performed by means of multivariate analysis.

When authentic chemical standards are not available, they can be manufactured. Because different enzymes are involved in the biogenesis of specific steroids, dedicated enzymatic reactions could be used to biosynthesize steroid standards for comparison with unknown features. In the absence of authentic standards or synthesized compounds, the identification process requires time-consuming and complex supplementary examinations of the MS/MS spectra and other physiochemical properties of the putative biomarkers. Consequently, identifying steroids is still the greatest challenge for steroidomics, and further progress is needed to achieve a high rate of identification.

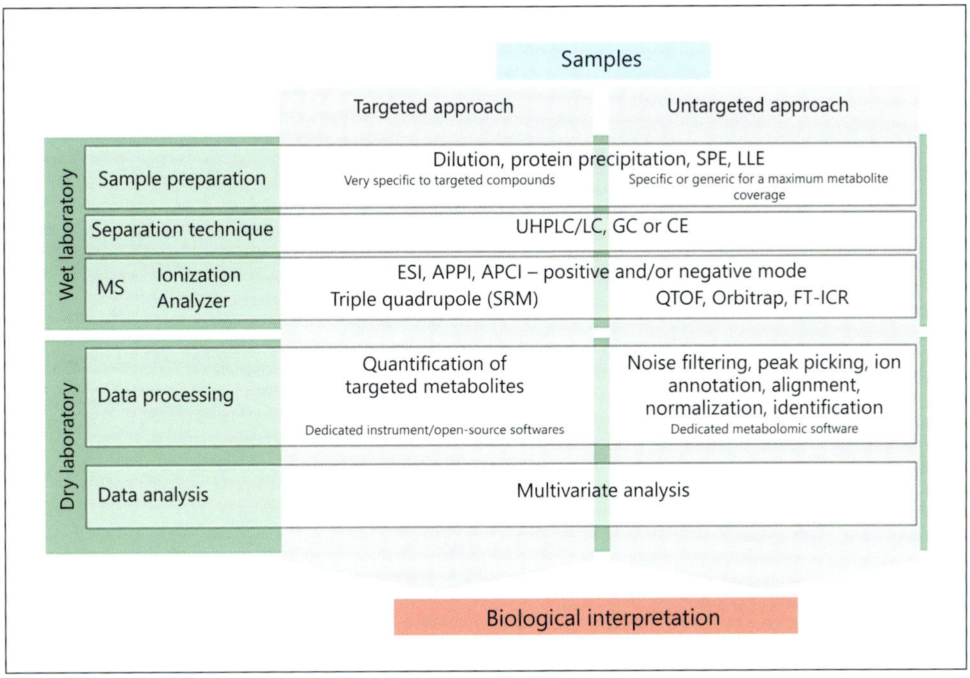

Fig. 3. Proposed steroidomic workflow (Jeanneret et al. [18]). SPE = Solid-phase extraction.

In doping control, this steroidomic workflow was followed by Boccard et al. [20] to discover and identify new steroid metabolites with the goal of improving the performance of existing testing procedures to detect T misuse. With that intention in mind, a controlled elimination study was performed on urine samples collected from subjects who had ingested T undecanoate. After dedicated solid-phase extraction of glucuro- and sulfo-conjugated steroids, all samples were analyzed by UHPLC-QTOF/MS^E.

QTOF-MS coupled to MS^E acquisition includes two functions: the first at low collision energy and the second with a collision energy ramp. This provides parent and fragment mass information in a single run, which is useful for both untargeted analyses and targeted metabolite profiling studies. Once these analyses were performed, a steroid database was applied for signal filtering, and orthogonal partial least-square discriminant analysis was performed on the resultant dataset to highlight the most relevant features (fig. 4). From the 436 steroid-related ion features provided by the UHPLC-QTOF/MS^E platform, a subset of 24 putative biomarkers was selected based on their contributions to the predictive component across all volunteers (fig. 4b).

By comparisons of exact masses and retention times with those of pure standards injected under the same conditions, ten of these compounds could be identified as known steroid phase II metabolites. All other relevant ions were assigned, based on their exact masses, to putative steroid-related compounds. In a series of six isobaric

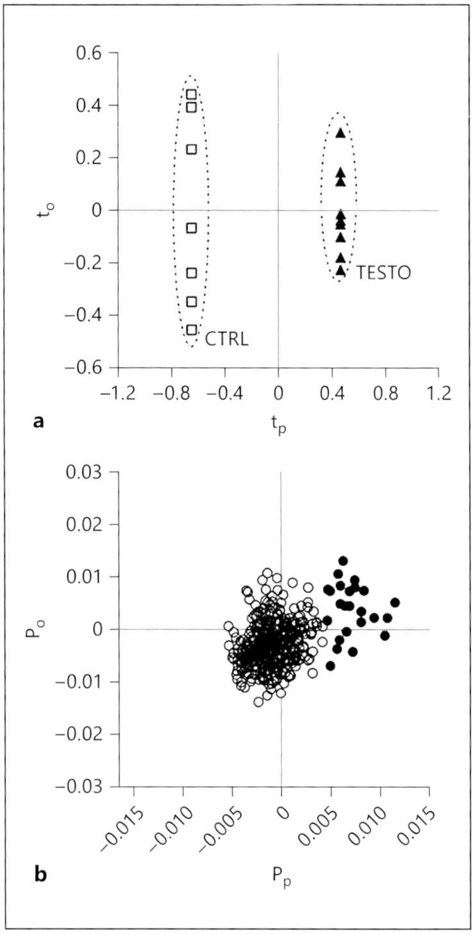

Fig. 4. Untargeted consensus orthogonal partial least square discriminant analysis model (Boccard et al. [20]). **a** Score plot. Sampling time points of the control group (CTRL) are symbolized by white squares and time points of the treated class (TESTO) by black triangles. **b** Loading plot. Unknown metabolites are symbolized by circles with nonrelevant compounds in white circles and putative biomarkers in black.

ions, corresponding to *m/z* 481.2438, the top-ranked candidate biomarker was potentially related to 6- or 16-hydroxyandrosterone glucuronide or Etio glucuronide. Even if further investigations must be performed to achieve unequivocal identification of all relevant features, identification of these candidate compounds further reinforces the feasibility of increasing actual detection ability (provided by T/E glucuronide in urine) and prolonging the traceability of T undecanoate misuse by using hydroxylated metabolites.

Although all doping controls for steroid abuse are currently performed on urine samples, Ponzetto et al. [21] recently generated the first example of a blood ‘steroid profile’ to confirm the hypothesis that steroid analysis in this matrix represents a complementary strategy to the current urine testing methods. For this purpose, 11 steroid hormones were quantified by UHPLC-MS/MS in serum samples obtained from a clinical study of T administration. After quantification, a multiway data analysis applied to the resultant dataset highlighted T and dihydrotestosterone as the most relevant biomarkers of T intake. Longitudinal follow-up of these two compounds was able to detect T abuse especially in cases involving individuals devoid of the UGT2B17 enzyme (responsible for T glucuronidation) and for transdermal application, two of the most troubling circumstances to confront in the context of routine urinary follow-up. Furthermore, blood matrix has a lower risk of manipulation and/or contamination than urine, and it can be assumed that for compounds circulating in the blood, the dose-concentration profiles can be accurately estimated for pharmacokinetic interpretation.

This work demonstrated that the discovery of new biomarkers of EAAS misuse should focus not only on urine, but also on blood matrix. For this purpose, the steroidomic approach has already been shown to be a powerful tool. In this context, a major effort should be made to improve identification procedures, as their application at the end of the workflow represents a crucial step in the path to biomarker discovery.

Circulating MicroRNAs: New Potential Biomarkers

One major challenge in the anti-doping field is the identification of specific and sensitive noninvasive biomarkers that can be routinely measured in easily accessible samples. A particularly promising class of biomarkers is miRNAs; these small (22-nucleotide) non-protein-encoding RNAs posttranscriptionally regulate gene expression via suppression of specific target mRNAs. Since their discovery in the early 1990s, miRNAs have been shown to play important regulatory roles in a wide range of biological and pathological processes [22].

In 2008, miRNAs were identified in serum, plasma, urine, saliva, and other body fluids. Although RNA molecules are generally unstable, circulating miRNAs are very stable and readily detectable. The mechanisms underlying the remarkable stability of miRNAs circulating in the blood have been intensively studied and debated [23]. Emerging evidence demonstrates that miRNAs in serum remain stable after being subjected to severe conditions that would degrade most other miRNAs. Despite the presence of RNase activity in plasma, subjecting plasma samples to up to 8 freeze-thaw cycles or incubating them at room temperature for up to 24 h has only a minimal effect on measured circulating miRNA levels [24]. By contrast, synthetic miRNAs added directly to plasma are degraded rapidly, suggesting that endogenous circulating miRNAs exist in a form that is resistant to plasma RNase activity [24]. Differential centrifugation and size exclusion chromatography experiments identified two populations of miRNAs in the blood: most circulating miRNAs cofractionate with complexes containing the Argonaute 2 protein, whereas a specific minority are predominantly associated with vesicles and high-density lipoprotein (fig. 5) [25, 26]. Both types of circulating miRNAs are sensitive to protease treatment of plasma, but are protected against digestion by plasma RNase [26]. The identification of extracellular Argonaute 2-miRNA complexes in plasma raises the

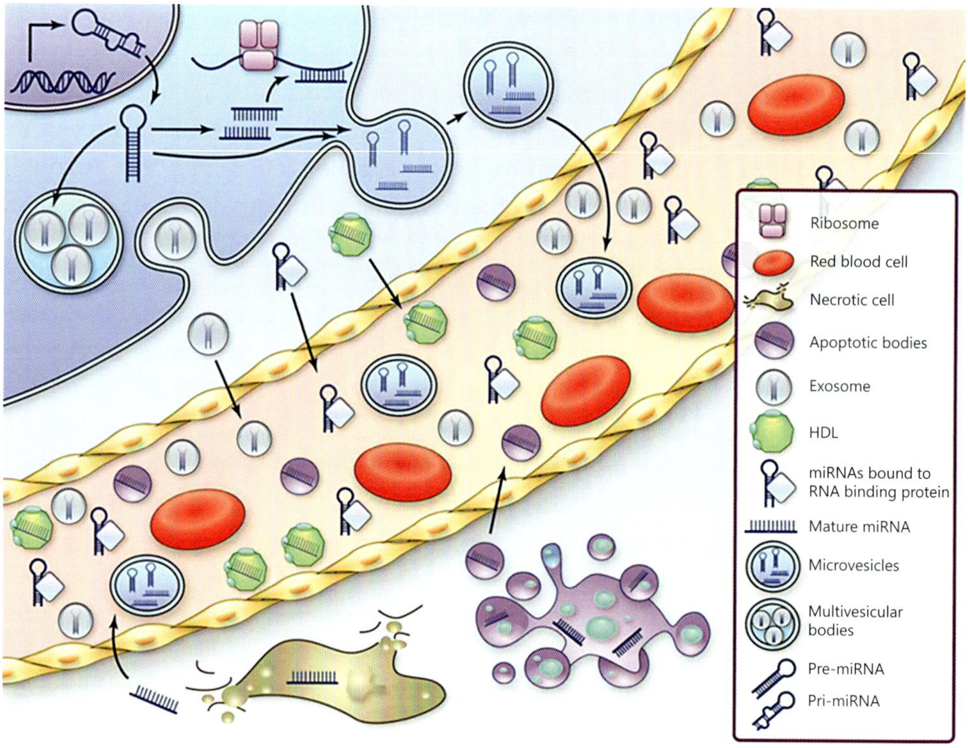

Fig. 5. Putative sources of circulating miRNAs. Circulating miRNAs may originate from apoptotic or necrotic cells, secretory vesicles such as exosomes or microvesicles (Kumarswami et al. [23]). HDL = High-density lipoprotein.

possibility that cells release functional miRNA-induced silencing complexes into the blood.

In the same way that certain biomarkers are used to detect the biological fingerprints of disease, other biomarkers can be used to detect the biological fingerprints of doping. The potential use of circulating miRNAs as specific biomarkers in the anti-doping field has been demonstrated by different laboratories. One recent study showed that a single injection of continuous erythropoietin receptor activator induces an increase in the plasma level of miR-144 [27], which plays an essential role in erythropoiesis in a number of organisms. This finding emphasized the potential use of miRNAs as circulating biomarkers for the detection of erythropoiesis-stimulating agents. In addition, Kelly et al. [28] identified 4 miRNAs that are differentially expressed between individuals receiving therapeutic replacement doses of recombinant human GH and normal controls or individuals with naturally high levels of GH, suggesting that circulating miRNAs could be used to detect recombinant human GH abuse. Furthermore, Leuenberger et al. [29] demonstrated that circulating miRNAs can also be used to detect autologous blood transfusions; the results of this study showed that transfusion of autologous blood triggered increases in the plasma levels of several miRNAs.

The use of circulating miRNAs to detect performance-enhancing agents could also be extrapolated to other doping trends, such as T abuse. Currently, the gold standard for detecting exogenous T administration is GC-MS analyses of urine samples, as described previously. At the Swiss Laboratory for Doping Analyses, however, measurements of circulating miRNAs in plasma and serum are used to detect T abuse, and preliminary results show that longitudinal measurements of miRNA levels in plasma represent a promising approach. The use of circulating miRNAs to detect blood doping could be incorporated into the adaptive model of the ABP [30]. As noted above, one of the advantages of miRNAs as biomarkers is their high stability in blood. In addition, in contrast to other hematological parameters, the levels of circulating miRNAs are not affected by environmental factors such as inadequate storage during transport of the blood samples, obviating the requirement for cumbersome documentation regarding sample transport and storage. Blood samples included in the hematological modules of the ABP are analyzed in laboratories accredited by WADA, and strict quality control criteria are applied to ensure that these analyses are executed according to forensic standards. Blood parameter analyses are performed using automated blood cell counters, and the resulting hematologic variables could be correlated to quantitative PCR measurements of circulating miRNA levels. PCR-based detection of miRNAs is a well-established, robust, and reproducible method with a number of key advantages, including its high sensitivity and specificity, potential for target multiplexing, and low RNA input requirements, all of which facilitate expression analyses, even in samples collected for anti-doping purposes with limited amounts of material. In addition, this technology has already been implemented in a large number of diagnostic laboratories, and routine protocols are well established. Quality controls could easily be included at every step to monitor sample hemolysis as well as extraction, RT, and quantitative PCR efficiencies, and these controls could be used as normalization factors. The incorporation of quality controls would help to eliminate within-subject variation and increase the efficiency and accuracy of evaluation of biological data.

References

1 Erotokritou-Mulligan I, Holt RI, Sönksen PH: Growth hormone doping: a review. Open Access J Sports Med 2011;2:99–111.

2 Saugy M, Cardis C, Schweizer C, Veuthey JL, Rivier L: Detection of human growth hormone doping in urine: out of competition tests are necessary. J Chromatogr B Biomed Appl 1996;687:201–211.

3 Dall R, Longobardi S, Ehrnborg C, Keay N, Rosén T, Jørgensen JO, Cuneo RC, Boroujedi MA, Cittadini A, Napoli R, Christiansen JS, Bengtsson BA, Sacca L, Baxter RC, Basset EE, Sönksen PH: The effect of four weeks of supraphysiological growth hormone administration on the insulin-like growth factor axis in women and men. GH-2000 Study Group. J Clin Endocrinol Metab 2000;85:4193–4200.

4 Wallace JD, Cuneo RC, Lundberg PA, Rosén T, Jørgensen JO, Longobardi S, Keay N, Sacca L, Christiansen JS, Bengtsson BA, Sönksen PH: Responses of markers of bone and collagen turnover to exercise, growth hormone (GH) administration, and GH withdrawal in trained adult males. J Clin Endocrinol Metab 2000;85:124–133.
5 Wu Z, Bidlingmaier M, Dall R, Strasburger CJ: Detection of doping with human growth hormone. Lancet 1999;353:895.
6 Erotokritou-Mulligan I, Basset EE, Kniess A, Sönksen PH, Holt RI: Validation of the growth hormone (GH)-dependent marker method of detecting GH abuse in sport through the use of independent data sets. Growth Horm IGF Res 2007;17:416–423.
7 Bidlingmaier M, Suhr J, Ernst A, Wu Z, Keller A, Strasburger CJ, Bergmann A: High-sensitivity chemiluminescence immunoassays for detection of growth hormone doping in sports. Clin Chem 2009; 55:445–453.
8 Wu Z, Devany E, Balarini G, Junnila R, Bidlingmaier M, Strasburger CJ: Specific monoclonal antibodies and ultrasensitive immunoassays for 20K and 22K human growth hormone. Growth Horm IGF Res 2010;20:239–244.
9 Voss SC, Robinson N, Alsayrafi M, Bourdon PC, Schumacher YO, Saugy M, Giraud S: The effect of a period of intense exercise on the marker approach to detect growth hormone doping in sports. Drug Test Anal 2014;6:582–586.
10 Holt RI, Böhning W, Guha N, Bartlett C, Cowan DA, Giraud S, Bassett EE, Sönksen PH, Böhning D: The development of decision limits for the GH-2000 detection methodology using additional insulin-like growth factor-I and amino-terminal pro-peptide of type III collagen assays. Drug Test Anal 2015;7:745–755.
11 Robinson N, Dollé G, Garnier PY, Saugy M: 2011 IAAF World Championship in Daegu: blood tests for all athletes in the framework of the Athlete Biological Passport. Bioanalysis 2012;4:1633–1643.
12 Donike M: Steroid profile in Cologne; in Donike M, Geyer H, Gotzmann A, et al (eds): Proceedings of the 10th Cologne Workshop on Dope Analysis, 7th to 12th June 1992. Cologne, Sport und Buch Strausse, 1993, p 47.
13 World Anti-Doping Agency. WADA Technical Document – TD2004EAAS: Reporting and Evaluation Guidance for Testosterone, Epitestosterone, T/E Ratio and Other Endogenous Steroids. 2004, http://www.wada-ama.org (accessed December 8, 2015).
14 Kuuranne T, Saugy M, Baume N: Confounding factors and genetic polymorphism in the evaluation of individual steroid profiling. Br J Sports Med 2014;48: 848–855.
15 World Anti-Doping Agency: WADA Technical Document – TD2016EAAS: Endogenous Anabolic Androgenic Steroids: Measurement and Reporting. 2016, http://www.wada-ama.org (accessed January 11, 2016).
16 Dominguez-Romero JC, Garcia-Reyes JF, Lara-Ortega FJ, Molina-Diaz A: Screening and confirmation capabilities of liquid chromatography-time-of-flight mass spectrometry for the determination of 200 multiclass sport drugs in urine. Talanta 2015; 134:74–88.
17 Badoud F, Guillarme D, Boccard J, Grata E, Saugy M, Rudaz S, Veuthey JL: Analytical aspects in doping control: challenges and perspectives. Forensic Sci Int 2011;213:49–61.
18 Jeanneret F, Tonoli D, Rossier MF, Saugy M, Boccard J, Rudaz S: Evaluation of steroidomics by liquid chromatography hyphenated to mass spectrometry as a powerful analytical strategy for measuring human steroid perturbations. J Chromatogr A 2016; 1430:97–112.
19 Dunn WB, Erban A, Weber RJM, Creek DJ, Brown M, Breitling R, Hankemeier T, Goodacre R, Neumann S, Kopka J, Viant MR: Mass appeal: metabolite identification in mass spectrometry-focused untargeted metabolomics. Metabolomics 2015;9:S44–S66.
20 Boccard J, Badoud F, Jan N, Nicoli R, Schweizer C, Pralong F, Veuthey JL, Baume N, Rudaz S, Saugy M: Untargeted profiling of urinary steroid metabolites after testosterone ingestion: opening new perspectives for antidoping testing. Bioanalysis 2014;6:2523–2536.
21 Ponzetto F, Mehl F, Boccard J, Baume N, Rudaz S, Saugy M, Nicoli R: Longitudinal monitoring of endogenous steroids in human serum by UHPLC-MS/MS as a tool to detect testosterone abuse in sport. Anal Bioanal Chem 2016;408:705–719.
22 Krol J, Loedige I, Filipowicz W: The widespread regulation of microRNA biogenesis, function and decay. Nat Rev Genet 2010;11:597–610.
23 Kumarswami R, Thum T: Non-coding RNAs in Cardiac Remodeling and Heart Failure. Circ Res 2013; 113:676–689.
24 Mitchel PS, Parkin RK, Kroh EM, Fritz BR, Wyman SK, Pogosova-Agadjanayan EL, Peterson A, Noteboom J, O'Briant KC, Allen A, Lin DW, Urban N, Drescher CW, Knudsen BS, Stirewalt DL, Gentleman R, Vessella RL, Nelson PS, Martin DB, Tewari M: Circulating microRNAs as stable blood-based markers for cancer detection. Proc Natl Acad Sci U S A 2008;105:10513–10518.
25 Arroyo JD, Chevillet JR, Kroh EM, Ruf IK, Pritchard CC, Gibson DF, Mitchell PS, Bennett CF, Pogosova-Agadjanyan EL, Stirewalt DL, Tait JF, Tewari M: Argonaute2 complexes carry a population of circulating microRNAs independent of vesicles in human plasma. Proc Natl Acad Sci U S A 2011;108:5003–5008.

26 Chevillet JR, Kang Q, Ruf IK, Briggs HA, Voitech LN, Hughes SM, Cheng HH, Arroyo JD, Meredith EK, Gallichotte EN, Pogosova-Agadjanyan EL, Morrissey C, Stirewalt DL, Hladik F, Yu EY, Higano CS, Tewari M: Quantitative and stoichiometric analysis of the microRNA content of exosomes. Proc Natl Acad Sci U S A 2014;111:14888–14893.
27 Leuenberger N, Jan N, Pradervand S, Robinson N, Saugy M: Circulating microRNAs as long-term biomarkers for the detection of erythropoiesis-stimulating agent abuse. Drug Test Anal 2011;3:771–776.
28 Kelly BN, Haverstick DM, Lee JK, Thorner MO, Vance ML, Xin W, Bruns DE: Circulating microRNA as a biomarker of human growth hormone administration to patients. Drug Test Anal 2014;6:234–238.
29 Leuenberger N, Schumacher YO, Pradervand S, Sander T, Saugy M, Pottgiesser T: Circulating microRNAs as biomarkers for detection of autologous blood transfusion. PLoS One 2013;8:e66309.
30 Leuenberger N, Robinson N, Saugy M: Circulating miRNAs: a new generation of anti-doping biomarkers. Anal Bioanal Chem 2013;405:9617–9623.

Federico Ponzetto
Swiss Laboratory for Doping Analyses
Chemin des Croisettes 22
CH–1066 Epalinges (Switzerland)
E-Mail federico.ponzetto@chuv.ch

Author Index

Subject Index